INTRODUCTION TO FOOD TOXICOLOGY

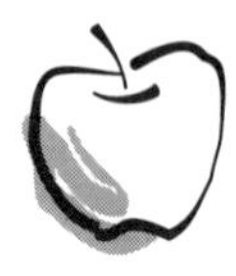

FOOD SCIENCE AND TECHNOLOGY

International Series

A complete list of the books in this series appears at the end of this volume.

INTRODUCTION TO FOOD TOXICOLOGY

Takayuki Shibamoto

Department of Environmental Toxicology
University of California, Davis
Davis, California

Leonard F. Bjeldanes

Department of Nutritional Sciences
University of California, Berkeley
Berkeley, California

ACADEMIC PRESS, INC.
Harcourt Brace & Company
San Diego New York Boston London Sydney Tokyo Toronto

This book is printed on acid-free paper. 

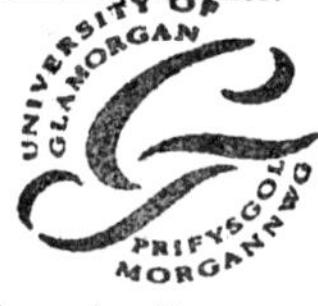

Academic Press, Inc.
1250 Sixth Avenue, San Diego, California 92101-4311

United Kingdom Edition published by
Academic Press Limited
24–28 Oval Road, London NW1 7DX

Library of Congress Cataloging-in-Publication Data

Shibamoto, Takayuki
Introduction to food toxicology. / Takayuki Shibamoto, Leonard F. Bjeldanes.
p. cm. – (Food science and technology)
Includes index.
ISBN 0-12-640025-3
1. Food–Toxicology. I. Bjeldanes, Leonard F. II. Title.
III. Series.
RA1258.S55 1993
615.9'54–dc20

92-41626
CIP

PRINTED IN THE UNITED STATES OF AMERICA
93 94 95 96 97 98 MM 9 8 7 6 5 4 3 2 1

Contents

CHAPTER 3

Biotransformation

CHAPTER 4

Natural Toxins in Animal Foodstuffs

CHAPTER 5

Natural Toxins in Plant Foodstuffs

CHAPTER 6

Fungal Toxins Occurring in Foods

CHAPTER 7

Toxic Food Contaminants from Industrial Wastes

CHAPTER 8

Pesticide Residues in Foods

CHAPTER 9

Food Additives

Foreword

The field of toxicology is rapidly expanding in scope and relevance, and consequently formal academic programs encompassing teaching, training, research, and outreach are increasing. The toxicology program at U.C. Davis represents one of the pioneering programs that is experiencing a surge in student enrollments at both the undergraduate and the graduate levels. This development is welcome because the appropriate education at all levels is important to meet the growing demand for toxicologists. Graduates with a sound education in the principles of toxicology and industrial hygiene are increasingly needed to deal with environmental, industrial, agricultural, and food safety issues with respect to toxic and potentially toxic chemicals. Trained professionals are critical to ensure development of rational legislation implementation of practical guidelines, and human and environmental health and safety.

The field of food toxicology has developed rapidly as a popular area of study in several universities and colleges. The field, which has evolved from food science, food safety, pesticide chemistry, and toxicology, represents a broad area requiring a strong scientific base in physical, chemical, mathematical, and biological sciences and an appreciation for food chemistry, natural products, analytical chemistry, pharmacokinetics, risk assessment, and some legal orientation. Because of the broad scope of toxicology it is imperative that students study the relevant disciplines and synthesize them into a coherent framework that will ensure a solid professional base. In this regard this textbook provides an excellent comprehensive treatment of the important subjects, principles, and concepts of food toxicology. Toxicology, risk assessment, pesticides, microbial toxins, food additives, and naturally occurring poisons are covered in a manner providing the undergraduate, and the lay reader, with a clearly written, well-organized, basic treatment of these topics.

The study of food toxicology is a very appropriate field for undergraduate science majors. It gives graduates a solid background in sciences and it can be applied to the study of important everyday phenomena and common consumer products. This textbook will be of benefit to the field and greatly appreciated by students, formal and informal, of food toxicology.

John E. Kinsella

Preface

Food is one of the most essential materials for the survival of living organisms, following perhaps only oxygen and water in importance. People have been learning how to prepare appropriate foods since prehistoric times. However, there was probably a tremendous sacrifice of human lives before people learned to find and prepare safe foods. For thousands of years trial and error was the only method to detect the presence of poisons in certain foods. Systematic data on poisons in foods have been recorded for only approximately 200 years or so. Moreover, only a decade has passed since food toxicology was first taught in universities.

This textbook is aimed at students who do not have strong backgrounds in either toxicology or food science. The format is designed primarily to teach students basic toxicology; toxicants and their fates in foods and the human body are then discussed.

The number of students who are interested in toxicology has increased dramatically in the past several years. Issues related to toxic materials have received more and more attention from the public. The issues and potential problems are reported almost daily by the mass media, including television, newspapers, and magazines. Major misunderstandings and confusion raised by those reports are almost always due to lack of basic knowledge about toxicology among consumers. This textbook provides the basic principles of food toxicology in order to help the general public better understand the real problems of toxic materials in foods.

Takayuki Shibamoto

CHAPTER 1

Principles of Toxicology

Toxicology may be defined as the study of the adverse effects of chemicals on living organisms. Its historical origins may be traced to the time when our prehistoric ancestors attempted to eat a variety of substances in order to obtain adequate food. By observing which substances could satisfy hunger without producing illness or death, ancient people developed dietary habits which allowed for the survival and growth of the species. In its modern context, toxicology draws heavily on knowledge in chemical and biological fields and seeks a detailed understanding of toxic effects. Much of toxicology today involves studies of the effects of specific substances on specific biological and chemical mechanisms.

One of the fundamental concepts of toxicology is that the dose determines the toxicity. As noted by Paracelsus (1493–1541), "All substances are poisons; there is none which is not a poison. The right dose differentiates the poison from a remedy." Thus, the answer to the question, "Is this substance toxic?" must always be, "Yes, if taken in a large enough dose." Thus, two of the primary objectives of toxicology are to quantitate and to interpret the toxicity of substances.

I. Dose–Response

Since there are both toxic and nontoxic doses for any substance, we may also inquire about the effects of intermediate doses. In fact, the intensity of biological response is proportional to the dose of the substance to which the organism is subjected. Thus, as the dose of a substance approaches the toxic level, there is no one point at which all of the organisms in the group will suddenly develop toxic symptoms. Instead, there will be a range of doses to which individuals in the test group respond in similar ways.

Once the response has been properly defined, information from dose–response experiments can be presented in several ways. A frequency–response plot (Figure 1.1) is generated by plotting the percentage of individuals with a specific defined response as a function of the dose. If a range of doses of a particular hypertensive agent is administered to a group of patients, there will be a certain number of low doses where none of the patients will yield a specific response, which in this example could be a blood pressure of 140/100. The highest of these doses without the response is the "no-observed-effect level" (NOEL) indicated in Figure 1.1. As the dose is increased, the percentage of individuals responding with the 140/100 blood pressure will increase until a dose group where the maximum number of individuals within the group responds with this blood pressure. This dose, determined statistically, is the mean dose for eliciting the defined response in the population under study. As the concentration or dose of the hypothetical hypertensive agent is further increased, the individuals previously responding with the defined blood pressure will develop yet higher blood pressures. Eventu-

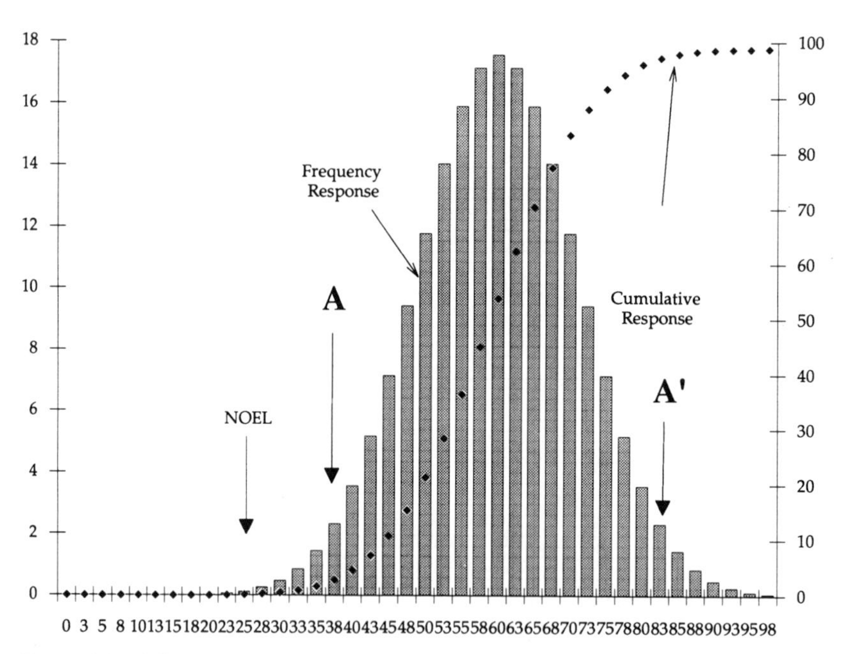

Figure 1.1 A frequency–response plot.

ally a dose will be reached at which all the patients within the test population respond with blood pressures higher than the defined level.

The curve that is generated by these data has the form of the normal Gaussian distribution, and therefore the data are subject to the statistical laws of such distributions. In this model, the numbers of individuals on either side of the mean are equal and the area under the curve represents the total population of individuals tested. The area under the curve bounded by lines from the inflection points (indicated A and A′) include the number of individuals responding to the mean dose plus or minus 2 SD from the mean dose, or 95.5% of the population. This mean value is useful in specifying a dose range over which most individuals respond in the same way.

Frequency–response curves may be generated from any set of toxicological data where a quantifiable response is measured simply by recording the percentage of subjects that responded at each dose minus the percentage that responded at the lower dose. Generally, the frequency–response curve obtained by experiment only approaches the shape of a true Gaussian distribution. Such curves illustrate clearly, however, that there is a mean dose where the greatest percentage of individuals will respond in a specific way. There will always be individuals who require either greater or smaller doses than the mean to elicit the same response. Individuals responding to smaller doses are called hypersensitive and individuals responding to greater doses are called hyposensitive.

Dose–response data and, in particular, information concerning the acute toxicity of substances are often presented as cumulative response vs. dose. In this case, various doses of the substance are administered to groups of individuals and the percentage of individuals responding in a specific way is noted. In the case of a lethal response, the number of individuals that died is noted. In the case of a nonterminal response, such as modification of blood pressure, the number of individuals responding in each group with at least a certain specified blood pressure is noted. Prior experiments establish the broad range of doses over which the response of interest occurs. Data are plotted as a cumulative percentage of individuals responding in the desired manner vs. dose (Figure 1.1). Again, a range of doses too small to elicit a response is administered to establish the NOEL. As the dose increases, the percentage of responding individuals in each test group continues to increase until a dose is reached beyond which 100% of the individuals in the test group will respond.

The shapes of the cumulative–response curves are generally sigmoidal with a nearly linear portion at intermediate dose ranges. The mean toxic dose, or in the case of the lethal effect, the LD_{50}, is established from such curves (Figure 1.2). The LD_1 and LD_{99} are determined in like

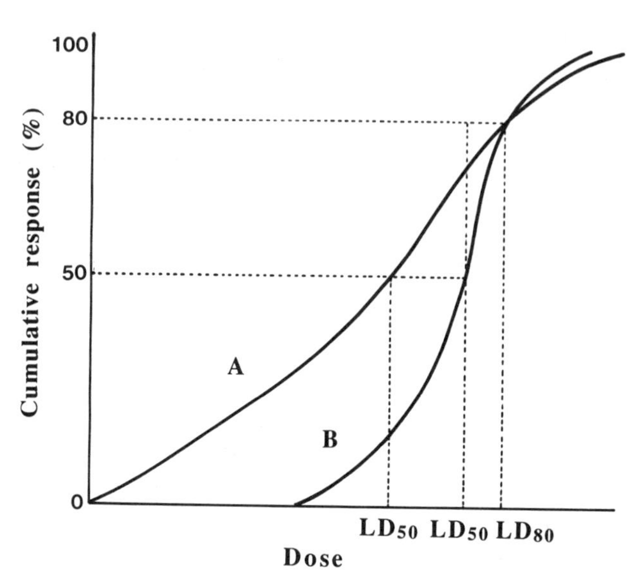

Figure 1.2 A typical cumulative–response curve for two different compounds.

manner. The slopes of the linear portions of these curves for different substances need not be in the same and the relative toxicities of these substances depend on the dose. These hypothetical compounds have the same LD_{80} and, therefore, have the same level of toxicity at this dose. However, below this dose compound A produces greater percentages of effect than compound B and in this dose range, therefore, is more toxic than compound B. At higher doses, however, compound B produces higher percentages of toxicity and, therefore, is more toxic than compound A. Based on LD_{50} information alone, compound A is more toxic than compound B. In comparing the toxicity of two substances the toxic response must be clearly defined, the dose range of toxicity must be indicated, and the slopes of the dose response curves must be compared.

The LD_{50} is a statistically determined value and represents the best estimation of the dose required to produce death in 50% of the organisms tested. The LD_{50} value should consequently always be accompanied by some means of estimating the error in the value. The probability range, or *p* value, which is most commonly used, is generally accepted to be less than 0.05. This value indicates that the same LD_{50} value would be obtained in 95 out of 100 repetitions of the experiment.

Although every substance will exhibit a lethal dose–response curve, there are wide differences in the LD_{50}'s for various substances. For example, the LD_{50} of caffeine is estimated to be about 200 mg/kg body weight; the LD_{50} of botulinum toxin, one of the most toxic substances known, is estimated to be about 100 ng/kg. On the other side of the scale, the LD_{50} of sodium chloride is estimated to be about 40 g/kg. As a general rule, substances with LD_{50}'s of 1 mg or less are considered extremely toxic. Substances with LD_{50}'s in the range of 1–50 mg/kg are in the highly toxic range. Moderate toxicity is ascribed to substances with LD_{50}'s in the range of 50–500 mg/kg. Substances with higher LD_{50}'s than this are generally considered to be nontoxic since relatively large amounts of material must be consumed in order to produce toxicity. For example, a substance with an LD_{50} of 2 g/kg requires consumption of about one cup of the material to produce toxicity in an adult human. On the other hand, extremely toxic substances with LD_{50}'s in the 1 mg/kg range require consumption of only drops to produce toxicity in an adult human.

II. Safety

Safety is defined as freedom from danger, injury, or damage. Absolute safety of a substance cannot be proven since proof of safety is based on negative evidence, that is, the lack of harm or the lack of damage caused by the substance. A large number of experiments can be run that may build confidence but still not prove the safety of a particular substance. Statistically, there is always the chance that the next experiment might show that the substance is unsafe. Our concept of safety has evolved over the years, and initially a substance was probably considered safe if it could be consumed without causing immediate death or acute injury. Our knowledge of toxic effects and our ability to test them have increased to the point where we now consider a substance relatively safe if it causes no adverse effects on specific biological systems. Today, certain substances are considered unsafe (or at least suspect) if they do nothing more than cause a change in the activity of a specific enzyme.

Since absolute safety cannot be proven, we must talk in terms of relative safety, and the conditions by which we evaluate safety must be carefully defined. Once the toxic effects in a species and the experimental conditions of toxicity testing have been carefully defined, relative toxicity of substances can often be indicated simply by measurements of lethal-dose curves and comparison of LD_{50}'s. Often, however, a more useful concept is the comparison of doses of the substance that elicit desired or undesired effects. For practical purposes, the margin of safety of a substance is considered to be large if the dose range between desirable and undesirable effects is large. If the desirable and undesirable dose ranges overlap each other, the margin of safety is small and considerable hazard is attendant on the use of such a substance.

The therapeutic index (TI) has been developed as a concept to quantify the margin of safety of a given substance. The TI is the ratio of dose required to yield a toxic effect (TD) to the dose required to yield a desired effect (the effective dose, ED), $TI = TDx/EDy$ (see Figure 1.3). Similar dose ratios may be used to compare toxic effects of two different substances or different toxic effects of the same substance. The median doses (TD_{50}, ED_{50}) are most commonly used for evaluation of the TI, but they can be useless when the two curves are not parallel. A more useful margin of safety can be determined by using the lower-percentage toxic doses (TD_1) and the higher-percentage effective doses (ED_{99}).

For food additives, the margin of safety, or dose ratio (roughly corresponding to the TI), has been arbitrarily set at 100. The toxic dose in the equation has been redefined as the NOEL and the effective dose is

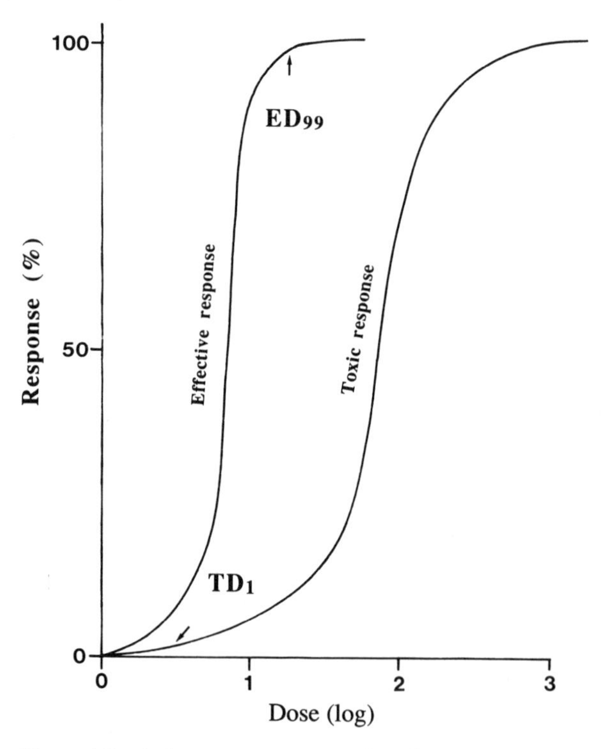

Figure 1.3 A dose–response curve for effective response and toxic response.

generally considered to be the minimum amount required to give the desired effect in a food, such as a particular color or taste. In other words, exposure to a food additive can be no greater than 1/100 of the highest dose that causes no adverse effect.

III. Absorption

In order for a substance to gain access to a specific effector site within an organelle of a complex organism, the substance must pass through a series of membranes. Although membranes in various parts of an organism have certain characteristics which distinguish them from one another, the basic compositions of the membranes are considered to be very similar. The currently accepted membrane model is illustrated in Figure 1.4. In this model, the membrane is represented as a phospholipid bilayer with a hydrophilic outer portion and a lipophilic inner portion. Proteins are dispersed throughout the membrane with some proteins transversing its entire width and projecting beyond both surfaces. The basic cell membrane is approximately 78-100 Å thick and is elastic. It is composed almost entirely of proteins and lipids with only small quantities of carbohydrate on the surface.

Substances cross the cell membrane by two major processes: diffusion (i.e., free, random movement of substances caused by kinetic motion) and active transport (i.e., movement of substances in chemical combination with carrier substances in the membrane). Most lipid-soluble xenobiotics

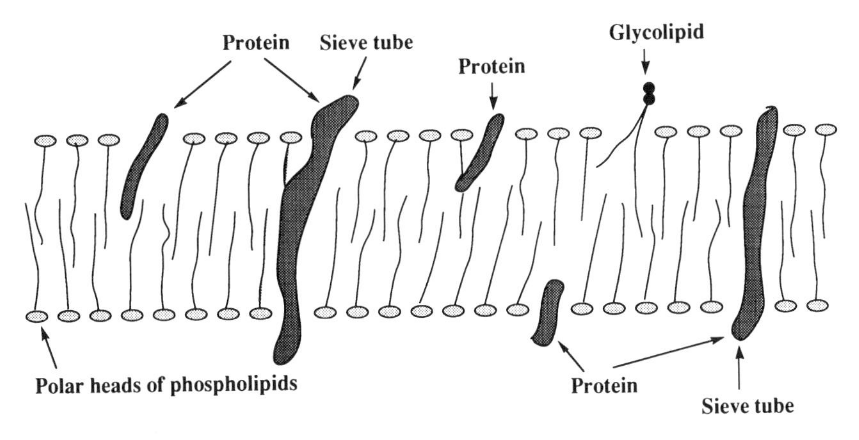

Figure 1.4 Model of membrane structure.

(foreign substances) are transported across membranes by simple diffusion within the lipid bilayer. Water, many dissolved ions, and certain water-soluble substances of smaller molecular weight diffuse through the aqueous pores in the cell membrane. These pores appear to be minute round holes approximately 8 Å in diameter with total area approximately 1/1600 of the total surface area of the cell. They are formed by the presence of large proteins that interrupt the membrane structure and extend through the membrane, thus providing direct aqueous passage through the interstices of the protein molecules. Despite their very small total area, these pores allow very rapid trans–membrane diffusion of water–soluble substances with a molecular mass less than about 100 Da. Although diffusion (whether through the lipid bilayer or through pores) is a very important process for transport of substances across membranes, it is not effective against a concentration gradient. Thus, the net result of simple diffusion processes is the elimination of transmembrane concentration differences. Net concentration differences can be developed or maintained, however, if pH or binding site differentials exist on either side of the membrane. This aspect will be discussed in more detail later as it relates to absorption from the gastrointestinal tract.

Many substances, such as nutrients, are moved effectively across membranes and against concentration gradients by active transport. Active transport is generally thought to involve the combination of the exogenous component with a protein carrier in the cell membrane. These protein carriers are specific for certain substances. Once the substance and the protein combine, the carrier complex moves through the membrane, where it separates at the inside surface and the substance is released. The carrier protein then returns to the outer portion of the membrane to combine with more exogenous compounds.

Several types of carrier systems exist in cell membranes, each of which transports only certain substances. One carrier system, for example, transports sodium to the outside of the membrane and transports potassium to the inside. Another carrier system actively transports sugars through the membranes of the intestinal and renal cells, while still other specific carrier systems transport different amino acids.

There is no specialized system that exists in mammals for the sole purpose of absorption of toxic agents as a group. These substances cross cell membranes by the same routes that desirable components cross the membranes. Diffusion, however, rather than active transport, is considered the primary mode by which toxicants enter an organism. For food-borne substances, the alimentary tract is the primary site of absorption, and for the absorption of substances which are highly lipid soluble, the mouth is the usual site.

There is a reasonable correlation between lipid solubility vs. water solubility of certain well-known alkaloids and their absorption following sublingual (oral) dosing. For cocaine, a substance which shows relatively high lipid solubility, the ratio of sublingual dose to subcutaneous dose is roughly 2 : 1 (twice as much required orally as under the skin) to produce the same response. On the other hand, morphine, a substance which shows relatively poor lipid solubility, requires a sublingual dose roughly 10 times that of the subcutaneous dose to give similar effects. These results are consistent with the major role of the lipid-diffusion process in the absorption of these alkaloids.

The stomach is an absorption site for certain substances depending on the extent to which they are uncharged in the relatively high acidity of the stomach. Weak acids, for example, are more lipid-soluble in their nonionized form in the stomach; they (as well as certain neutral substances) are absorbed into the lipid membrane, allowing them to diffuse into the circulating blood. Since the pH of the circulating blood is higher than the pH of the stomach, these acids are deprotonated to the ionized form and thus show a decreased tendency to penetrate the stomach wall. However, absorption in the stomach is not simply a matter of pH, for the presence of food generally tends to decrease the rate of absorption of most substances in the stomach regardless of their acid properties.

During absorption in the small intestine (the principal site of absorption of nutrients and non-nutrients alike), the charge characteristics of a substance again play the primary role in the rate of its absorption. Since the pH in the small intestine is close to neutral, strong acids and bases there will tend to have a charge. As a result, they tend to be absorbed to a lesser degree in the small intestine than neutral substances. However, unless the pK_a is very large or very small, there is a significant percentage of the substance in the neutral or nonionized form. Since the small intestine has a great area of absorption, absorption of acids and bases in this tissue can be nearly complete even though the charge equilibrium lies heavily in favor of the charged species.

Results of studies with steroids and certain derivatives of steroids have shown that the lipid solubility of these substances is important in their absorption. The lipid/water partition coefficients of certain steroids correlates highly with their absorption rates in the small intestine. The presence of polar components such as hydroxyl groups, leads to decreased lipid solubility and decreased rates of absorption.

Absorption in the small intestine, compared to that in the large intestine is relatively poor. However, the small intestine can serve as a site of absorption for certain substances, especially those produced by bacterial fermentation within the gut, or those which are highly lipid-soluble.

Although non-specific absorption of substances through lipid membranes occurs primarily in the alimentary tract, a few relatively toxic substances are absorbed by the active transport systems in the gut. For example, lead is absorbed by the system that normally transports calcium. Cobalt and manganese are absorbed by the iron-transport system. As stated previously, however, most toxicants are not subject to active transport.

Since the lipid solubility of a substance plays a primary role in determining its rate of absorption across the lipid membrane, the presence of binding sites on one side of the membrane and individual differences in certain membranes must also be considered. If a substance is selectively removed from solution by a component which binds to it, the amount of this material on one side of the membrane can increase greatly relative to the side where there are no binding sites.

Plasma albumin plays an important role in binding many foreign chemicals in the blood. The extent of binding depends primarily on the chemical characteristics of the substance and generally involves ionic interactions and hydrogen bonding. This binding can lead to high effective concentrations of certain substances in the circulating fluid. Because of the reversible nature of the binding, this process can result in significant concentrations of substances at remote sites in the organism.

Significant differences in permeability of various membranes for absorption of certain substances are often the result of differences in the pore sizes of these various membranes. For example, the pore sizes of tissue membranes in glomerular membranes are relatively large compared to those of membranes in other tissues. As a result, substances the size of small proteins can pass through the membranes of the glomerulus.

In comparison, absorption of certain types of substances into brain tissue relative to absorption into other tissues is greatly retarded. The term blood–brain barrier has been coined to account for this decreased absorption. The cause of the low permeability of the blood–brain barrier to certain substances is due to the manner in which cells of the capillaries are joined to each other. The membranes of adjacent cells are essentially fused with each other rather than having spaces between them. This double-thick membrane retards passage of substances through pores since passage by this route would require lining up of the pores of two adjacent capillaries. It has also been postulated that the presence of glial cells around the neural capillaries also serves to decrease the rate of absorption of certain substances. There is some controversy about this explanation, however, since there are sufficient openings between the glial cells to allow almost normal diffusion of fluid between the capillary blood and interstitial fluid in the brain tissue. The relative lack of protein in the interstitial fluid of the nervous tissue is another feature which appears to play a role in the decreased absorption of certain substances across the blood–brain barrier. This would provide decreased binding sites for certain types of substances in nervous tissue relative to other tissues in the body.

In effect, the blood–brain barrier results from the increased thickness of lipid tissue between the circulating blood and the nervous system, and it is very effective in excluding certain water-soluble substances from nervous tissue. Conversely, however, it is also effective in concentrating certain lipid-soluble substances within the brain. It has also been suggested that the blood–brain barrier serves as a sink for certain substances such as lead and mercury. The administration of these toxic substances leads to a buildup of levels in the blood-brain barrier tissues that results in decreased levels in the cerebral spinal fluid and nervous blood system. Although this effect would appear to protect against toxicity of these substances, their buildup in the blood–brain barrier tissues inhibits the transport of certain required nutrients into the central nervous system.

IV. Translocation

Translocation, or interorgan movement of substances in the body fluids, is governed by properties of various membranes and binding within the fluid. In addition, the extent of blood perfusion plays an important role in translocation of substances within the organism. Blood flow to various organs and tissues varies widely within the body. Total blood flow is greatest in the liver, kidney, muscle, brain, and skin and is much less in the fat and bone. Thus, in the absence of other characteristics such as selective absorption and specific tissue binding based on solubility, those organs with the greatest blood flow would be expected to contain the greatest amount of translocated substances. Certain other organs, such as the adrenals and thyroid, although having a small total volume of blood, have a relatively high flow of blood based on weight of total tissue. Thus, these organs would be expected to have higher concentrations of certain substances than would be expected on the basis of total blood volume.

In an adult human, the approximately 38 liters of body water is composed of three fluids: interstitial fluid (11 liters), plasma fluid (3 liters), and intracellular fluid (24 liters). By determining the apparent volume in which a substance appears to be dissolved, known as the apparent volume of distribution (Vd), some idea of the distribution of a substance throughout the body fluids can be obtained. Vd is the amount of toxin in the body/concentration of toxin in plasma. If the Vd appears to be small (less than 5 liters, for example) it is reasonable to suggest that the substance is confined to the plasma. Much lower plasma concentrations following administration of a substance and consequently much larger Vd's would indicate that the substance is probably distributed in the larger pool of body fluid and not confined to the plasma. Because of factors such as binding in specific tissues, the concentration of certain substances can be very low in plasma fluid following administration. The Vd for these types of substances would be extremely large, much larger than the total body fluid.

V. Storage

When the binding interactions of a substance with various components of the cells are sufficiently strong, the substance can remain associated with these components for extended periods. Under these circumstances these components of the body are said to be storage sites. The tendency for storage of various substances in the body depends on the chemical properties of the compound. The more polar, organic substances tend to be bound to protein in the blood or in the soft tissue, whereas inorganic substances with chemical properties similar to those of calcium tend to be stored in the bone tissue. Fatty tissues serve as sinks for absorption of most lipid-soluble materials.

Protein binding of various exogenous substances is well known and plays an important role in increasing the concentration of certain components at several sites of the body. Binding of substances to serum albumin is a common phenomenon. Collagen, the chief protein in the body, binds many ions, including calcium, barium, magnesium, strontium, beryllium, lead, arsenic, and mercury. Bone stores inorganics and is thus a particularly important storage site for inorganic ions; it is, for example, the principal storage site for lead and strontium.

In addition to these general body storage sites, organs such as the liver and kidney tend to concentrate and retain certain substances. Although it is not entirely clear which mechanisms are involved in maintaining the increased concentration of substances in kidney and liver tissue, protein binding appears to play an important role. Ligandin, a protein prevalent in liver, has high binding affinities for organic acids, azodyes, and certain steroids.

Tissue storage has variable effects on toxicity of administered substances. The storage of a substance at a site distant from a site of toxicity can effectively reduce the toxicity of the material. For example, whereas lead is toxic to erythrocytes and to certain organs, it is not toxic in the bone and is safely stored there. On the other hand, if a substance is stored at the site of toxicity, storage will increase the toxicity of the material. For example, storage in the bone of strontium-90, a radioactive isotope of strontium, serves to increase its half-life in the body and results in its increased toxicity in the bone.

An additional feature to be considered is that certain substances can displace others from storage sites. Thus, administration of one substance can result in toxic effects of another substance which had been previously administered. This displacement behavior has been observed repeatedly with certain drugs that are bound to plasma proteins. Conversely, a toxin is usually displaced from its site of action by a less toxic agent, resulting in decreased toxicity of the first substance. Also, when binding sites are eliminated, the substances which they contain can be introduced into the circulation in free form. This behavior has been seen with fat-soluble vitamin A. Rapid loss of fat in an individual who had been consuming relatively large amounts of vitamin A with no toxic effect resulted in symptoms of hypervitaminosis A. In this case, the fat stores had absorbed significant amounts of vitamin A and, with the rapid loss of weight, the vitamin A which they contained was released into the circulation.

VI. Excretion

Of the various routes by which toxic substances in the diet can be excreted from the body, urinary excretion is the most important. This applies to both the number of substances and the quantities of each substance excreted. Fecal excretion is important for substances that are either unabsorbed from the gastrointestinal tract or are secreted in the bile. In the maternal system, excretion of substances in milk plays a minor role in the removal of toxic agents. Certain drugs, certain pesticides, and toxic agents found in moldy food are excreted to a small extent in milk; however, this route of excretion is important in some cases because of the impact of these excreted substances on a nursing infant.

The kidney excretes toxicants via the same route as it excretes substances normally present in the body (Figure 1.5). Passive glomerular filtration is dependent upon the filtration rate and the degree of plasma protein binding. The glomerular capillaries have large pores (40 Å) and therefore all but the large molecular weight proteins are filtered at the glomerulus. Only toxicants that are significantly bound to these larger proteins are not filtered at the glomerulus.

A substance in the tubular urine may be excreted in the urine or it may be passively absorbed back into the bloodstream. Polar or water-soluble substances will tend not to be reabsorbed and will pass into the urine. However, the more lipid-soluble materials will tend to be passively reabsorbed through the tubular membranes. The acid–base properties of the substance play a significant role in the rates of passive secretion into the urine. Thus, acidic substances are most effectively excreted into less acidic urine. However, metabolic conversion of a weak acid to a

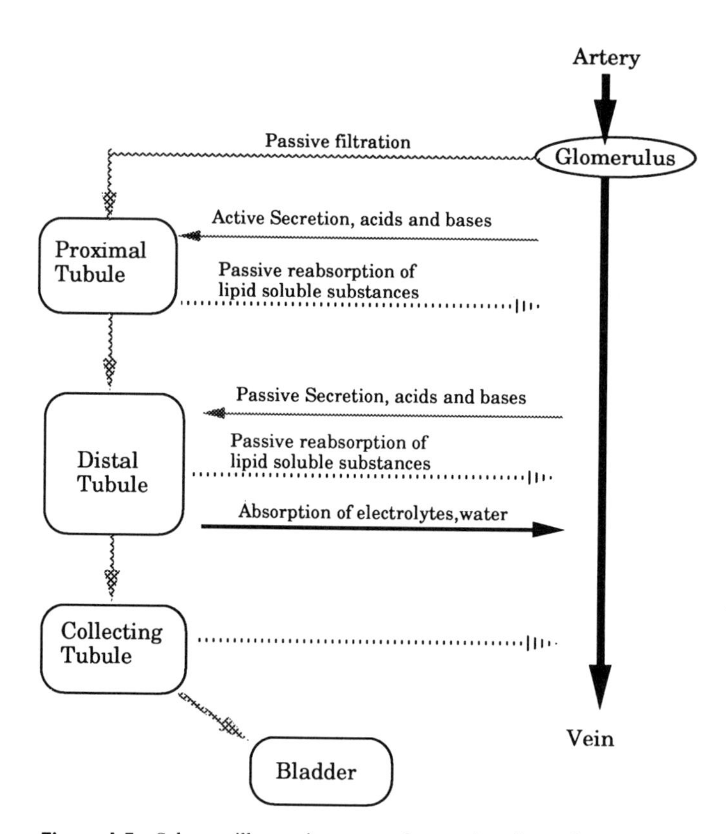

Figure 1.5 Scheme illustrating normal excretion from the kidney.

much stronger acid assures ionization of the substance in the tubule and therefore prevents reabsorption of the material, which leads to rapid excretion in the urine. Rates of excretion of weak organic bases are mainly affected by alteration in the pH of the urine, and excretion of weak bases is most efficient in more acidic urines.

Active tubular secretion also plays an important role in the excretion of certain substances into the urine. In the proximal renal tubule, strong organic acids and bases are added to the glomerular filtrate by active, carrier-mediated tubular secretion, while organic acids are transported by the system that secretes naturally occurring substances such as uric acid. Many organic bases are transported by another system that secretes choline and histamine, among other substances. Although protein binding of substances inhibits their excretion by the filtration route, protein binding does not inhibit excretion by this active role.

Since the sites for this active secretion are limited, various compounds can compete with one another for secretion. For example, substances that are transported by the organic-acid transport system can compete with uric acid for the specific excretion pathway, which can lead to gout due to an increase in plasma uric acid concentration. As another example, a substance known as probenecid (developed during World War II to decrease the rate of excretion of penicillin and, thereby, increase its plasma half-life) competes with penicillin for the acid transport system in the kidney.

Weak acids and bases undergo reabsorption or excretion in the proximal and distal tubules of the kidney by a process of passive diffusion that is relatively minor process compared to the mechanisms of renal excretion discussed previously. The importance of this process and the direction of net flow of materials depend on pH gradient and the acid properties of the substance. Under normal conditions, even when the pH gradient in the distal tubule favors diffusion into the urine, the net effect is reabsorption since the bulk of the compound will diffuse out of the urine as reabsorption of strong electrolyte and water creates a concentration gradient of the nonionized form in the direction of urine to blood. Under conditions where tubular urine is more alkaline than plasma, the acids are excreted more rapidly, primarily because of the decrease in the net passive reabsorption. Under conditions of more acid tubular urine, excretion of weak acids is reduced.

Urinary excretion and renal toxicity of substances can be influenced by the developmental stage of the organism. For instance, certain components of the kidney excretory system, such as the active transport system, are not fully developed in newborns. Thus, the clearance of certain organic acids is less efficient in a newborn than it is in an adult. This results in an increased toxicity of this type of substance in the newborn. On the other hand, some substances that are toxic to the adult are not toxic to the newborn because of this decreased capacity for active transport. Thus, for certain substances that are toxic to the kidney, decreased capacity for active transport would result in decreased concentration in the kidney and therefore decreased toxicity relative to toxicity in organisms where active transport is fully operative.

Although for many substances biliary excretion is of minor importance compared to urinary excretion, bile is a primary site of excretion of certain compounds and their metabolic products. The rate of bile formation is much less than the rate of urine formation. An important anatomical difference between the liver and the kidney is that the liver has a dual blood supply consisting of blood from the portal vein and the hepatic artery. The blood in the liver, unlike that in the kidney, circulates at a relatively slow rate, which allows ample time for lipid-soluble materials to penetrate liver cells and to be excreted in the bile.

Since blood from the intestines passes directly to the liver via the hepatic portal vein, the liver can play an essential role in removing many toxic substances from the blood before they reach the general circulation. However, since the bile drains directly into the small intestine, substances in the bile are either excreted in the feces or transformed by bacteria in the intestines into a form which is reabsorbed. In the latter case, a cycle known as the enterohepatic cycle (Figure 1.6) can be set up which can considerably increase the time a substance is in the body.

Although little is known about the mechanisms of biliary excretion, evidence indicates that a passive diffusion process is operative for certain substances. For example, the concentrations of certain metal substances such as mercury and cadmium are the same in the bile as in the plasma. There is also evidence for an active transport system leading to considerably increased concentrations of substances in the bile relative to the plasma. Such a mechanism appears to be operative for lead and arsenic. In addition, there is evidence for three separate systems for active transport of organic compounds into the bile based on their acidic, basic, or neutral properties.

The synthetic hormone diethylstilbestrol (DES) is an example of the potential importance of biliary excretion. DES is normally eliminated only via biliary excretion and is subject to extensive enterohepatic circulation. Preventing biliary excretion of DES by bile duct ligation greatly increases its half-life in the body and increases its toxicity by about 130-fold.

Bile production and biliary excretion of many substances have been shown to be influenced by substances, such as phenobarbital, that induce the microsomal enzyme system to produce enzymes, which increase bile

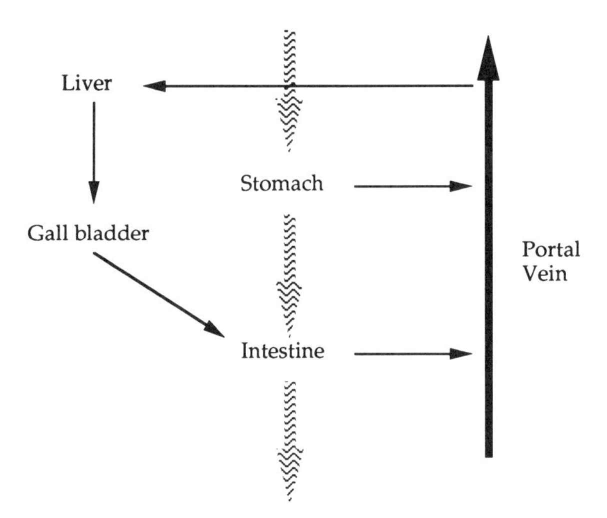

Figure 1.6 The enterohepatic cycle.

flow and excretion of certain substances. It is reasonable to suggest that natural components of the diet may influence the activity of the liver in this way as well.

Suggestions for Further Reading

1. Clark, W. G., Brater, D. C., and Johnson, A. R. (1988). "Goth's Medical Pharmacology," 12th Ed. Mosby, St. Louis.
2. Guyton, A. C. (1976). "Textbook of Medical Physiology," 5th Ed. W. B. Saunders, Philadelphia.
3. Hayes, A. W. (1989). "Principles and Methods of Toxicology," 2nd Ed. Raven Press, New York.
4. Hodgson, E., and Levi, P. E. (1987). "A Textbook of Modern Toxicology," Elsevier, New York.
5. Klaassen, C. D., Amdur, M. O., and Doull, J. (1986). The basic science of poisons. *In* "Toxicology" (L. J. Casarett and J. Doull, eds.), 3rd Ed. Macmillan, New York.
6. Loomis, T. A. (1978). "Essentials of Toxicology," 3rd Ed. Lea and Febiger, Philadelphia.

CHAPTER **2**

Determination of Toxicants in Foods

Food safety assessment depends upon the determination of toxic materials in foods. It is important to develop accurate analytical methods to interpret the data correctly.

The major tasks of chemical analysis in food toxicology involve separating a toxicant from other chemicals and then determining the amount. Almost by definition, toxicants are present in very low levels because substances with any significant level of any toxicant are rejected as foods. This is illustrated by the fact that a distaste for a particular food is developed after it is associated with an episode of illness.

To provide a system for toxicity testing which can be relied upon to give state-of-the-art assessments of toxicity while also minimizing the numbers of animals used as well as cost and time requirements, so-called decision-tree approaches have been proposed. A decision-tree protocol for testing the safety of food components has been proposed by the Scientific Committee of the Food Safety Council in the United States. Although details of the protocol are likely to be modified, the overall scheme has received strong support from the scientific community. A summary of the decision-tree protocol proposed by the Food Safety Council is presented in Figure 2.1.

The initial phase of this protocol is the proper identification of the substance to be tested. In the case of pure substances, this is a relatively simple matter since procedures for chemical identification and criteria for purity are well established. However, determination of safety of complex mixtures is more complicated. In these cases, it is ultimately desirable to establish the composition of the mixture and to determine which components of the mixture are responsible for biological activity. In lieu

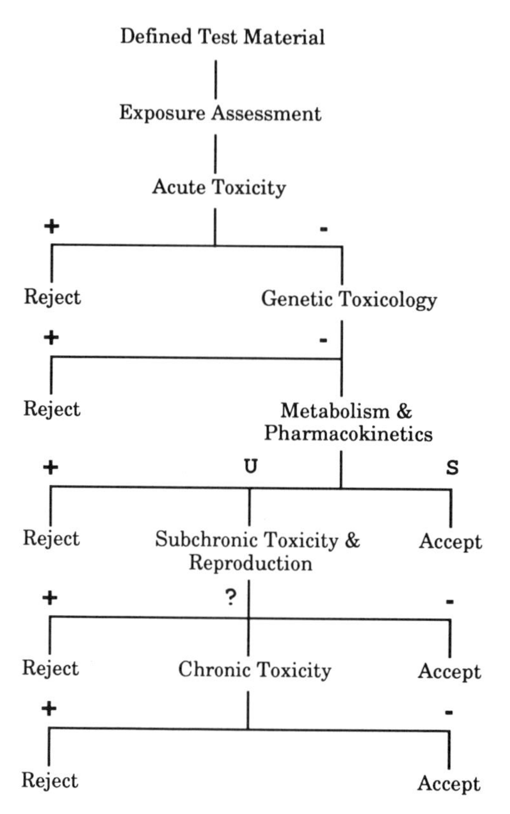

Figure 2.1 Summary of decision-tree protocol proposed by U.S. Food Safety Council. +, presents a socially unacceptable risk; −, does not present a socially unacceptable risk; S, metabolites known and safe; U, metabolites unknown or of doubtful safety; ?, decision requires more evidence.

of detailed information on the composition of a mixture, however, the process by which it is obtained must be described in as much detail as possible so that the test material can be reproduced in other laboratories.

I. Qualitative and Quantitative Analyses of Toxicants in Foods

The qualitative and quantitative analyses of toxicants in foods are the principal tasks of food toxicology. When toxicity is discovered in a food, the analyst's first job is to identify the toxic material(s) in the food. The analysis of toxicants requires both an assay for detecting the poison and a method for separating it from the rest of the chemicals in the food. The assay for detecting the poison is usually the toxic effect that has been observed. Since it is rarely desirable to use humans, a "model system" must be selected (usually rats or mice) to use in the identification process.

The food is first separated into its components and each component is tested for toxicity. The active fraction is further separated and tested—and this continues until the pure toxicant can be completely isolated. At this point the structure of compound can be identified by chemical analysis.

The method of elucidating the structure of unknown chemicals has dramatically improved since the development of analytical instruments such as ultraviolet spectroscopy (UV), infrared spectroscopy (IR), nuclear resonance spectroscopy (NMR), and mass spectroscopy (MS).

Once a toxic chemical has been identified, the quantitative analysis can be accomplished with a chemical analysis designed specifically for that chemical. In order to allow legally binding conclusions about toxicant levels in foods, the U.S. government monitors a set of approved methods which have a certain set of criteria about quality. For example, unless circumstances warrant, the recovery by the method must be at least 80%. Additionally, certain physical processes are required when preparing the testing samples.

II. Sample Preparations for Determination of Toxicants

A. Sampling

Although a toxicant found in any food is significant, one of the purposes of using chemical analysis is to determine the amount of a toxicant and the probability of overexposure. To accomplish this, samples used for analyses must be taken according to a design. Well-developed statistical methods are usually employed that are relevant to the types of conclusions sought. It is helpful, for example, to take replicates at different points within the population to discover the variation. However, this variation should not be confused with the error that occurs within the analytical method.

Samples might be collected for a screen of a certain class of compounds, but sample treatments required by different compounds may be contradictory and make a "total screen" impossible. For some chemicals, the sample might need to be treated with base in the field to prevent acid breakdown, while other chemicals might require an acid treatment to prevent base breakdown. In some cases, a general screen test may be desired in order to probe for a family of chemicals, and from that point the samples are often collected again, and then treated and analyzed specifically for chemicals discovered in the screen.

B. Extraction

Once a representative sample of suitable size has been selected, the next step in analysis is usually to separate the analyte from the matrix. The ability of a specific analytical technique to detect a particular analyte is as dependent on the percent of chemical recovered by the method as it is on the sensitivity of the detector at the end of the process. Since all parts of the food sample need to be equally exposed to the extraction, it is often necessary to blend or chop the sample so that it is homogeneous. The food can then be dissolved and the fibers and coarse insoluble materials filtered away.

Organic chemicals have varying degrees of water solubility, from organic acids like vinegar that are polar to the organic oils that are nonpolar and float in a separate layer on top of water. When a nonpolar organic phase is mixed with an aqueous phase the two will separate into distinct layers. So many of the organic solvents are nonpolar that the term "organic phase" is used as equivalent to the nonpolar or "oil layer" in such a mixture. The molecules that may be insoluble in water and that thereby dissolve in the organic phase, as well as those that may be slightly soluble in water but have a greater affinity to the organic phase, will migrate into the organic layer. This one step can yield a great deal of separation from the matrix if a nonpolar analyte is extracted from a polar matrix such as fruit, or in the opposite case, if nonpolar material such as fatty tissue is to be cleaned away from a polar analyte.

There can be many different types of organic phases, as well as interactions with organics (such as acetone) that pass between the phases and affect the relative solubility of the molecule of interest in each phase. Hence, solvent choice is a crucial factor in extraction. The important factors for solvent choice are as follows:

1. Good solubility for the target chemicals
2. High purity (no additional contamination)

3. Low boiling point (easy to remove)
4. Low cost (large amount of solvent is often required)
5. Low toxicity

If the analyte has an acidic or basic group that might be charged at one pH and neutral at some other, it is the neutral molecule and therefore the pH at that point that will facilitate the movement of most of the chemical to the organic phase. The addition of salt can also increase the polarity of the water phase and drive solvents like acetone and chemicals that were associating with them into the water from the water phase. These differences can allow fine tuning of extraction methods so that molecules that are less polar than the analyte can be cleaned off in one step. The analyte can then be brought out by changing conditions to drive it into the organic phase.

C. Cleanup

After an extraction, any further separation of the analyte from the matrix before placing the sample on the final analytical device is called cleanup. The term comes from the need to minimize the amount of extraneous chemicals placed on the sensitive analytical devices to keep the injection ports and columns clean for as long as possible. Cleanup is a preparative step in an analytical method. A preparative separation is designed to yield some chemical sample for further use, while an analytical separation is designed to quantitate the target analyte. Most cleanup methods are chromatographic separations optimized for complete recovery of the analyte with less resolution of chemicals in the mixture.

D. Chromatography

Chromatography is an elegant method of chemical separation that, using only a few simple principles, has given chemists tools for separating and purifying practically all chemicals. Because of its simplicity, efficiency, and wide range of applications, chromatography has had a great impact on chemical toxicology.

This separation principle in chromatography is based on a mobile phase and a stationary phase. The mobile phase contains a mixture of chemicals, one of which is the target analyte. When the mobile phase moves through the stationary phase, the chemicals will have a tendency to move more slowly than the mobile phase because of their affinity for the stationary phase. The different affinities for the stationary phase will cause them to slow at different rates, and this will separate them in the mobile phase.

The great diversity and power of the method derive from the many types of mobile phases (many solvents and properties of the solvents, as well as gas as a mobile phase and the gases and temperature of the gas) and the great variety of stationary phases (varying from silica, paper, and gel to nonpolar, oil-like stationary phases).

III. Toxicity Testing

A. Preliminary Steps for Toxicity Testing

Another important step in the initial phase of safety assessment is to estimate the levels of the substance to which the population is exposed. One method for making such an estimate is based on a dietary survey in which individual consumers are interviewed to obtain information on the types of foods they consume. Another method is market basket analysis in which food is purchased from retail outlets, prepared by typical methods, and then analyzed for the components in question. Per capita disappearance of a particular food component is computed by dividing the annual domestic production plus import quantities by the number of people in the country.

Once the identity of the test substance has been carefully defined and the levels of exposure have been estimated, priorities for biological testing are established. Purified substances or mixtures with well-defined characteristics for which estimates of exposure are the greatest will generally have the highest priority for further testing. Considerations of chemical structure may also be involved in the priorities assessment. Substances chemically related to known toxins are also likely to receive a high priority for subsequent testing.

B. Acute Toxicity

The first toxicity test to be run on the substance is generally the acute toxicity test in which the chemical is given to rats or mice, most commonly in a single dose. The toxic effects that occur within 24 hr of exposure are noted. The primary purpose of the acute toxicity test is to determine the level of the substance which induces mortality in laboratory animals. It is at this point in the testing protocol that median lethal dose (LD_{50}) is determined. Information obtained from these acute toxicity tests is generally used as a basis for establishing dose and route of exposure for subsequent prolonged toxicity tests. Except in the rare instance where the substance is found to be too acutely toxic to be considered for food use, the substance will be submitted for genetic toxicity testing and for studies of metabolism and pharmacokinetics.

C. Genetic Toxicity

The primary objective of genetic toxicity testing is to determine the tendency of the substance to induce mutations in the test organism. A mutation is an inheritable change in the genetic information of a cell. Approximately 10% of all human diseases may have a genetic component and thus may arise from a mutation of one form or another. It is well known, for example, that Down's syndrome, Kleinfelter's syndrome, sickle-cell anemia, and cystic fibrosis arise from specific genetic changes. Most if not all cancers are thought to have their origin in one or more mutations. Indeed, most substances (85–90%), except for hormones, that are carcinogenic in animal species have been shown to be mutagenic by one assay or another. Although much more information is required before the converse correlation can be established, the fact that a substance is shown to be mutagenic by appropriate tests places it under considerable suspicion as a possible carcinogen.

The decision-tree approach proposes a battery of genetic tests early in the testing scheme. It is suggested that a battery of tests can be developed that will yield a high degree of correlation between mutagenicity and carcinogenicity such that, based on the results of mutagen tests alone, a substance can be banned from use in food because of its carcinogenic probability. If the substance is not shown to be of high carcinogenic probability based on the results of this battery of tests, it must be submitted to further tests, perhaps including long-term carcinogenicity studies.

Although the details of an appropriate mutagenicity test battery are the subject of continuing controversy, the general outline seems to be fairly well established. Assays for which there seem to be general support include analyses of point mutations (localized changes in DNA) in microorganisms and in mammalian cells, investigation of chromosomal changes (major recombinations of genetic material) in cultured mammalian cells and in whole animals, and investigation of cell transformation (tumors produced by implantation in animals) using cultured human or other mammalian cells.

Perhaps the most widely used assay for point mutation employs specially constructed strains of *Salmonella typhimirium* mutants in which the pathway to histidine biosynthesis is blocked. This assay system, known as the Ames Assay, is used to detect reverse point mutations of the base-pair substitution or the frame-shift type. The organisms have been constructed with deficiencies in the DNA repair system and in the biosynthetic pathway for construction of the cell wall. In addition, certain bacterial strains carry antibiotic resistance that has been shown to increase sensitivity of these strains to certain types of mutagens. In order to mimic the mammalian metabolism of certain compounds, a tissue homogenate, most often from the liver, is incorporated into the test system. Before the tissue homogenate is prepared, donor animals are dosed with certain inducing agents, such as phenobarbital or Aroclor, to increase their rate of metabolism and the tendency to activate many mutagens.

In practice, the test organism and the substance to be tested are placed on a minimal glucose agar petri dish either with or without the inclusion of the tissue preparation, and then the petri dishes are incubated for the appropriate time. Since the petri dishes contain only minimal amounts of histidine, enough to allow only one or two divisions of the bacteria, colonies of bacteria will grow only after the occurrence of a mutation that produces histidine independence. The assay is flexible in that metabolic characteristics of many different animal species and many different tissues can be tested directly by the use of preparations from appropriate organs.

Another test which uses microbial organisms to determine mutagenic potential of a substance is known as the host-mediated assay. In this test a bacterial organism is injected into the peritoneal cavity of a mammal, usually a rat, and the animal is treated with the test substance. The test substance and its metabolites enter the circulation of the animal, including the peritoneal cavity. After an appropriate period, the test organism is removed from the peritoneal cavity and examined for induction of mutations.

A third mutagenesis assay, known as the dominant-lethal test, determines genetic changes in mammals. In this test males are treated with the test substance and mated with untreated females. The dominant-lethal mutation will arise in the sperm and can kill the zygote at any time during development. Females are dissected near the end of gestation and the numbers of fetal deaths and various other reproductive abnormalities are noted.

Assays for point mutations also have been developed using mammalian cell lines. One cell line that has been used extensively is the Chinese hamster ovary cell for which resistances to various substances such as 8-azaguanine are used as markers. In contrast to the *Salmonella* system, these Chinese hamster ovary cell lines detect mainly forward mutations. One problem often encountered with such assays is the variability in metabolic capability of the cell line. Thus, in some cases tissue homogenates such as those used in the Ames Assay are incorporated or the test cells are used in the host-mediated assay, as is most commonly done with bacterial cells.

Mutation of the more general type (those which are not point mutations) may be determined by scoring of induced chromatid and chromosomal aberrations. Structural changes in chromosomes may be caused by breaks in the chromosomal unit. If the two ends of the break remain separated, chromosomal material is lost, resulting in visible breaks in the chromosome.

The cell transformation assay, in which mammalian cells are used, is an important aspect of any battery of short-term genetic toxicity tests. Many cell lines have been developed for measurement of malignant transformation following exposure to a test substance. Embryo fibroblasts from rat, hamster, and mouse are commonly used cell lines. After a period of normal growth, cells are suspended in an appropriate buffer and treated with a test substance, and then portions of cells are tested for survival rates. The remaining material is plated out on an appropriate medium, and the transformed cells are observed at the colony stage. Malignancy of cells can be confirmed by the production of tumors following transplantation of transformed cells into the appropriate host.

If the genetic toxicology studies lead to the finding of mutagenesis, with the implication of possible carcinogenicity, a risk assessment is applied. If the substance is mutagenic in several assays that are correlated with human carcinogenesis and the intended use of the substance results in appreciably high human exposures, then with no further testing, the substance may be banned from further use. If the substance is determined to be of low mutagenic risk because, for example, it is mutagenic in several assays but only at very high doses or the mutagenic activity is observed in only one of the assays, then further studies must be conducted.

D. Metabolism

Metabolic studies would be conducted following the tests for mutagenesis. The objective of this phase of testing is to gain both a general and a quantitative understanding of the absorption, biotransformation, disposition (storage), and elimination characteristics of an ingested substance after a single dose and after repeated doses. If the biological effects of metabolites are known, the decision to accept or reject the substance can be made on this basis. For example, if all the metabolites can be accounted for and they are all known to be innocuous substances, then the test substance is considered safe. However, if certain metabolites are toxic or if much of the parent substance is retained within certain tissues, then further testing may be indicated. Further support for the potential hazard of a substance will be derived from the knowledge that metabolism in a test species, in which the substance has appreciable toxicity, is similar to the metabolism in humans. Thus, knowledge of the metabolism and pharmacokinetics of a substance is essential for establishing the relevance of results from animal testing to projecting likely hazards in humans.

E. Subchronic Toxicity

Based on the results of these initial investigations, subchronic toxicity studies may be designed. Subchronic tests generally are of several months' duration and may extend to 1 year. The objective of the subchronic studies is to determine possible cumulative effects on tissues or metabolic systems. Conventional subchronic studies designed to evaluate the safety of food components are generally limited to dietary exposure for 90 days in two laboratory species, one of which is a rodent. Subchronic tests generally include daily inspection of physical appearance and behavior of the test animal. Weekly records of body weight, food consumption, and characteristics of excreta are maintained. Periodic hematological and eye examinations are performed in addition to biochemical tests of blood and urine. Under certain circumstances, tests are run for hepatic, renal, and gastrointestinal functions along with measurements of blood pressure and body temperature. All animals are autopsied at the termination of the experiment and examined for gross pathologic changes, including changes in the weights of the major organs and glands.

F. Teratogenesis

Teratogenesis testing is an important aspect of subchronic testing. Teratogenesis may be defined as the initiation of developmental abnormalities at any time between zygote formation and postnatal maturation. Relatively little is known about the mechanisms of teratogenesis. It may be caused by radiation, a wide range of chemicals, dietary changes, infection, temperature extremes, or physical trauma. One cannot predict whether a specific substance will be teratogenic based on chemical structures. Because our knowledge of mechanisms of teratogenesis is relatively primitive, teratogenesis assays rely primarily on prolonged testing periods in animals. Administration of substances to bird embryos has been used with some success. However, since the embryos develop with no metabolic interchange with the outside environment, in contrast to the placenta-mediated interchange for mammalian embryos, teratogenesis testing in mammals is much preferred.

The phase of embryonic development most susceptible to adverse influences is organogenesis. As illustrated in Fig 2.2, the human fetus is most susceptible to anatomical defects at around 30 days of gestation. That is, exposure to a teratogenic influence around this period is most likely to produce anatomical defects in the developing fetus. One of the major problems in teratogenesis testing is that organisms may be susceptible to teratogenesis for only a few days during the growth of the fetus. If the test substances are not administered precisely at this time, the teratogenic effect will go undetected. Exposure to a teratogen prior to organogenesis may produce no effect or may lead to fetal death and no teratogenic response will be seen. Exposure to a teratogen following the period of organogenesis may lead to functional problems that may be relatively difficult to observe and may not be detected as teratogenic effects.

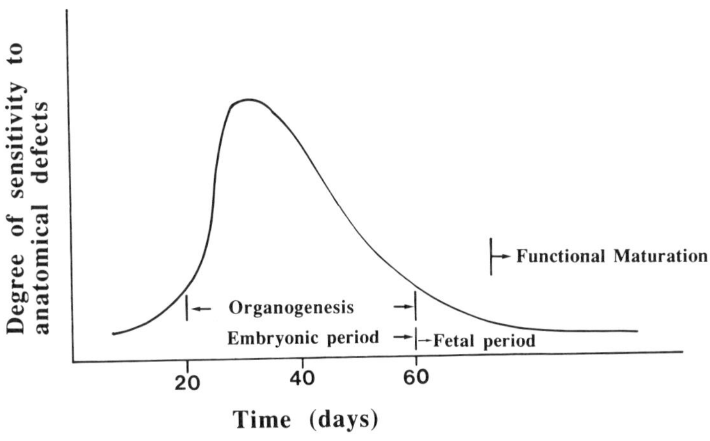

Figure 2.2 Degree of sensitivity of human fetuses to anatomical defects at various times during gestation.

Factors that determine the effective dose of the substance to which the fetus is exposed are (1) the efficiency of the maternal homeostatic processes, and (2) the rate of passage of a teratogen across the placenta. The maternal homeostatic processes depend on several factors, including the efficiency of liver metabolism and possible excretion of the substance into the bile, possible metabolism and urinary excretion by the kidney, and tissue storage and protein binding. These processes work together in the maternal system to reduce the overall concentration of the substance to which the developing fetus is exposed. The placenta can serve as an effective barrier to passage of certain water-soluble substances of large molecular weight into the fetal circulatory system. However, in the case of certain more lipid-soluble compounds (methylmercury, for example) the placenta does little to retard passage into the fetal system.

Teratogenesis testing protocols should include both short-term (1–2 days) treatments of pregnant females during organogenesis and continuous treatments during gestation. Teratogenesis tests that include short-term dosing avoid effects of maternal adaptive systems such as induction of metabolic pathways in the liver. This testing protocol also avoids preimplantation damage and increases the likelihood that the embryos will survive to the period of organogenesis. The continuous dosing protocol ensures that critical periods of organ development are covered and monitors cumulative effects both in the maternal and fetal systems. For example, it can monitor the changes in concentrations and composition of metabolites to which the fetus is exposed during gestation vis-a-vis the diminished metabolic activity of the maternal liver, or it can monitor the level of saturation of maternal storage sites in relation to a rise in the concentration of the test substance in the fetal system.

Since adverse effects on the reproductive system may arise from many causes, tests of reproductive toxicity may include treatment of males prior to mating, short-term dosage of females starting prior to mating and continuing on to lactation, short- and long-term dosing of females during the period of organogenesis and in other periods, and pre- and postnatal evaluation of the offspring. These tests can involve large numbers of animals and periods of time comparable to what would be required for carcinogenesis tests. As a result, measurement of reproductive toxicity can be a very time consuming and expensive procedure. Both mechanistic understanding and testing efficiency are sorely needed in this important area of toxicology.

Toxic effects observed in this battery of acute and subchronic tests are evaluated to determine if the tests are relevant to actual conditions of exposure. Many substances at this point in the testing procedure can be rejected from use if their toxicity is sufficiently high. On the other hand, a final decision to accept a relatively nontoxic substance cannot be made if the substance

1. is consumed at a substantial level,
2. possesses a chemical structure leading to a suspicion of carcinogenicity,
3. shows effects on subchronic toxicity testing that would suggest the possibility that long-term exposure would lead to increased toxicity, or
4. shows positive results in tests of genetic toxicity.

G. Chronic Toxicity

The general objective of chronic toxicity testing is to assess toxicity resulting from long-term, relatively low-level exposure which would not be evident in subchronic testing. Testing protocols require administration of the test substance by an appropriate route and in appropriate dosages for the major portion of the test animal's life.

Chronic toxicity tests are designed so that each treated and control group will include sufficient numbers of animals of both sexes of the chosen species and strain to have an adequate number of survivors at the end of the study for histopathological evaluation of tissues and for statistical treatment of the data. Selecting the proper size of the test group is a major problem in chronic toxicity tests. Table 2.1 indicates the required group sizes as determined by statistical theory. Large numbers of animals must be used if low percentage effects are to be detected. To reduce the numbers of animals required in theory to detect small percentage effects, protocols involving large doses are generally used. However, this practice is coming under increasing scrutiny since the test organism is likely to respond quite differently to high doses of the test

TABLE 2.1
Theoretical Sizes of Test Groups Required to Determine Toxicity at Indicated Frequencies and Level of Significance

True frequency of toxic effect	1 in 20		1 in 100	
Level of significance	0.05	0.001	0.05	0.001
Least number of animals for each dose	58	134	295	670

material than to low doses. For example, the rates of enzymatic processes such as absorption, excretion, metabolism, and DNA repair are highly sensitive to substrate concentration and are saturable. Thus, high doses of a substance may produce toxic effects by overwhelming a system that readily disposes of low doses. Research continues into the existence of a threshold dose below which exposure to a carcinogen may be safe. In the meantime, food-additive law in the United States has taken the prudent though much debated view that there is no safe dose of a carcinogen.

In most cancer tests, 50 animals of each sex are used for each dose level. Body weights are recorded periodically throughout the testing period, and the level of food consumption is monitored. Animals are examined for obvious tumors, and at the end of the experiment the animals are autopsied and subjected to detailed pathological examination.

Rats and mice are widely used in chronic testing because of their relatively low cost and the large volume of knowledge available concerning these animals. The strain of animals used for the test depends on the site of toxicity of the test substance and the general susceptibility of the strain to various toxic agents. Generally, strains with some known sensitivity to a range of carcinogens are used. It is likely that a carcinogenic effect will be shown in these animals if the substance is indeed carcinogenic.

Variations in diet can considerably complicate interpretation of the results from chronic toxicity testing. Administration of semi-synthetic diets can result in increased tumor yield with several types of carcinogens compared to experiments using unrefined diets. Diets that provide insufficient calories result in decreased tumor incidence while protein deficiency retards tumor growth. Dimethylaminoazobenzene-induced carcinogenesis is enhanced with riboflavin deficiency in rats. The influences of various dietary components on carcinogenesis are often complex and the mechanism of action is often specific to the carcinogen in question. Many dietary components, such as certain indoles, flavonoids, and certain pesticides that induce xenobiotic metabolizing systems in the liver and other tissues, will decrease the carcinogenic potency of many substances.

Even when due consideration is given to the various aspects of chronic toxicity testing mentioned in the previous discussion, several other more or less incidental factors can influence the outcome of such tests. For example, the temperature and humidity of the room in which the animals are housed must be carefully controlled, as must the type of bedding used in the cages. Cedar wood used as bedding has influenced the outcome of cancer testing, perhaps due to induction of xenobiotic metabolizing enzymes by volatiles from the cedar. Furthermore, cancer tests that are said to differ only with respect to the time of year during which they were performed have produced different results. Thus, it is necessary for even the most well-designed chronic toxicity tests that reproducibility of experimental results be determined.

The chronic toxicity test provides the final piece of biological information on which to base a decision to accept or reject a substance suggested for food use. If no carcinogenic effects are found, this information, along with all previous data, and the estimations of exposure are included in the overall risk assessment of a substance. If a substance is determined to be a carcinogen, then in most instances current U.S. law prohibits its use as a food additive. Further testing is needed only if some of the tests are considered faulty or if unexpected findings make the test design retrospectively inadequate to answer the questions raised.

Suggestions for Further Reading

1. Brusick, D. (1987). "Principles of Genetic Toxicology," 2nd Ed. Plenum Press, New York.
2. Calabrese, E. J. (1983). "Principles of Animal Extrapolation." Wiley, New York.
3. Campbell, T. C. (1980). Chemical carcinogens and human risk assessment. *Fed. Proc.* **39,** 2467.
4. Clayson, D. B., Krewski, D., and Munro, I. (eds.) (1985). "Toxicological Risk Assessment." CRC Press, Boca Raton, Florida.
5. Gad, S. C., and Chengelis, C. P. (1988). "Acute Toxicology Testing, Perspectives and Horizons." Telford Press, Caldwell, New Jersey.
6. Grice, H. E. (ed.) (1984). "The Selection of Doses in Chronic Toxicity/Carcinogenicity Studies." Springer-Verlag, New York.
7. Heddle, J. A. (ed.) (1982). "Mutagenicity: New Horizons in Genetic Toxicology." Academic Press, New York.
8. Kalter, H., and Warkany, J. (1983). Congenital malformations, part II. *N. Engl. J. Med.* **308,** 491.
9. Moutschen, J. (1985). "Introduction to Genetic Toxicology." Wiley, New York.
10. Newberne, P. M. (1975). Pathology: Studies of chronic toxicity and carcinogenicity. *J. Am. Assoc. Anal. Chem.* **58,** 650.
11. Poole, A., and Leslie, G. B. (1989). "A Practical Approach to Toxicological Investigations." Cambridge University Press, New York.
12. Tomatis, L. (1979). The predictive value of rodent carcinogenicity tests in the evaluation of human risks. *Annu. Rev. Pharmacol. Toxicol.* **19,** 511.
13. Wilson, J. G. (1975). Reproduction and teratogenesis: Current methods and suggested improvements. *J. Am. Assoc. Anal. Chem.* **58,** 657.
14. Zeise, L., Wilson, R., and Crouch, E. (1987). Dose-response relationships for carcinogens: A review. *Environ. Health Perspect.* **73,** 259.
15. Aurand, L. W., Woods, A. E. and Wells, M. R. (1987). "Food Composition and Analysis." Van Nostrand Reinhold, New York.
16. Ball, G. F. M. (1988). "Fat-Soluble Vitamin Assays in Food Analysis: A Comprehensive Review." Elsevier, New York.

17. Curry, A. S. (ed.) (1985). "Analytical Methods in Human Toxicology." Verlag Chemie: Weinheim, Deerfield Beach, Florida.
18. Egan, H., Kirk, R. S., and Sawyer, R. (1981). "Pearson's Chemical Analysis of Foods," 8th Ed. Churchill Livingstone, New York.
19. Pierson, M. D., and Stern, N. J. (eds.) (1986). "Foodborne Microorganisms and Their Toxins: Developing Methodology." Marcel Dekker, New York.
20. Willard, H. H., Merritt, L. L., Jr., Dean, J. A., and Settle, F. A., Jr. (1981). "Instrumental Methods of Analysis," 6th Ed. van Nostrand, New York.

CHAPTER **3**

Biotransformation

The construction of the cellular membrane confers on it a high degree of selectivity in absorption of most water-soluble or highly polar substances. This selectivity of absorption allows specific routes of uptake for certain water-soluble nutrients and provides a significant level of resistance to toxicity of most water-soluble substances. On the other hand, the very properties that allow for selectivity in absorption of water-soluble materials provide an almost completely nonselective uptake of lipid-soluble substances. Thus, although most living organisms are nearly impervious to certain unwanted water-soluble substances, and must expend energy to absorb required water-soluble substances, they are unable to prevent absorption of most lipid-soluble substances.

These features of living membranes result in pronounced differences between the potential toxicity of lipid- and water-soluble substances. A water-soluble toxin placed in the environment will eventually be distributed throughout the aqueous components of the environment. A lipid-soluble substance, however, even if it is placed in a large aqueous medium such as the ocean, is likely to be concentrated in living tissue by selective solubility in the living membranes.

I. Conversion of Lipid-Soluble Substances

Apparently in response to this tendency for lipid-soluble substances to penetrate cellular membranes, higher organisms have developed metabolic systems that convert lipid-soluble substances to more water-soluble metabolites. Most of the important reactions in the conversion of lipid-soluble substances to the more water-soluble form have been classified as either Phase I or Phase II reactions. Phase I reactions generally consist of oxidations, reductions, or hydrolysis. Phase II reactions generally involve reactions of an exogenous substance or Phase I metabolite with a highly polar endogenous substance. This process considerably increases the water solubility of the exogenous substance and thereby facilitates its excretion.

II. Phase I Reactions

Oxidation is perhaps the most important of the Phase I reactions. In general, these reactions are mediated by a cytochrome P450-containing enzyme system. This metabolic system, also known as the "mixed function oxidase system," requires NADPH as an initial electron donor and molecular oxygen as a formal oxidant (Figure 3.1). In the presence of NADPH and oxygen, the enzyme system transfers one atom of oxygen to the compound while another atom of oxygen is reduced to form water. The electron of NADPH is transferred to cytochrome P450 by the enzyme NADPH–cytochrome P450 reductase (Figure 3.1), also known as NADPH–cytochrome C reductase. The overall process combines a xenobiotic (i.e., foreign compound) with the oxidized form of cytochrome P450. This complex is reduced and combines with oxygen to form an

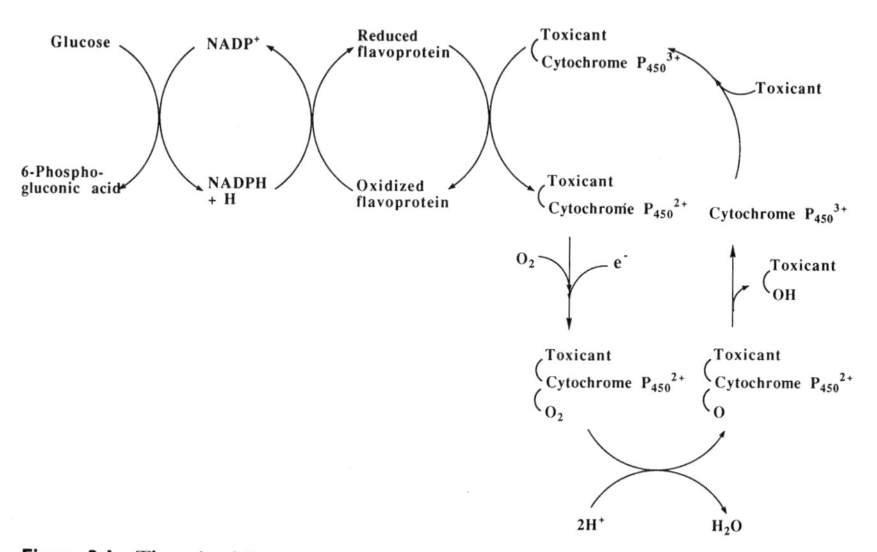

Figure 3.1 The mixed function oxidase system.

activated oxygen–xenobiotic–cytochrome complex. After a series of electron transfers, water, the oxidized form of cytochrome P450, and the oxidized xenobiotic are produced.

Although this oxidation system is found in many tissues in the body, the principal site of oxidation of most xenobiotics is in the smooth endoplasmic reticulum of the liver, and they can be isolated in the form of microsomes upon homogenization and centrifugation of a homogenate of liver tissue. There are many forms of cytochrome P450 with various specificities for certain substances.

In addition to mediating many oxidations, the cytochrome P450 electron transport system also mediates certain reductions such as the conversion of azo and aromatic nitro compounds to the corresponding amines.

Other important enzymes in the Phase I reactions of certain exogenous substances which are not involved in the cytochrome P450 system are epoxide hydrolase, certain esterases, and amine oxidase. Although amine oxidase can be isolated from the microsomal fraction, it has distinctly different specificities from the cytochrome P450 oxidation system. In general, the amine oxidase system preferentially metabolizes strong bases, whereas the cytochrome P450 system metabolizes weak bases. Epoxide hydrolase is another enzyme distant from the cytochrome P450 system but nonetheless important in the early stages of xenobiotic metabolism. Epoxide hydrolase mediates the addition of water to epoxides to form the trans-dihydrodiol and therefore plays an important role in the conversion of certain lipid-soluble substances to the more water-soluble diols. Many mammalian tissues also contain a wide variety of esterases and amidases. These enzymes mediate the addition of water to amide and ester bonds, resulting in the production of the corresponding acid and alcohol or amine. These products are then susceptible to certain Phase II conjugation reactions.

A further important group of Phase I reactions involves reduction of aldehydes and ketones. The required hydrogenases are present in many mammalian tissues, and the product alcohols can be either excreted or further conjugated by the Phase II processes. Examples of Phase I reactions are shown in Figures 3.2–3.15.

III. Phase II Reactions

A summary of the various Phase II reactions is shown in Figures 3.16 and 17. In Phase II reactions, the addition of a highly polar component to a previously oxidized or reduced substrate produces a highly polar

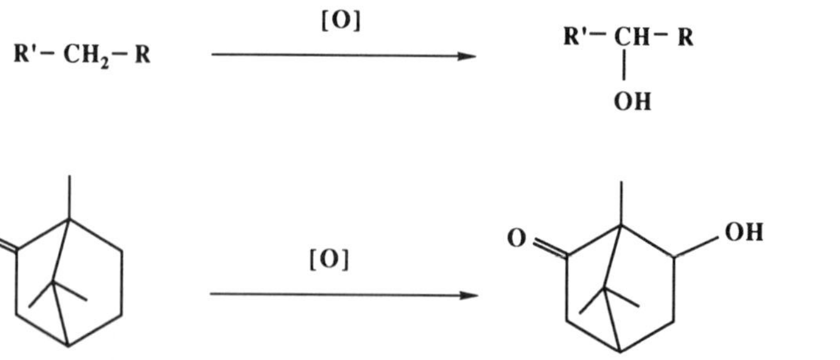

R'− CH$_2$− R —[O]→ R'− CH(OH)− R

Camphor —[O]→ 1-Hydroxycamphor

Figure 3.2 An oxidation process of Phase I reactions: aliphatic hydroxylation and a typical example.

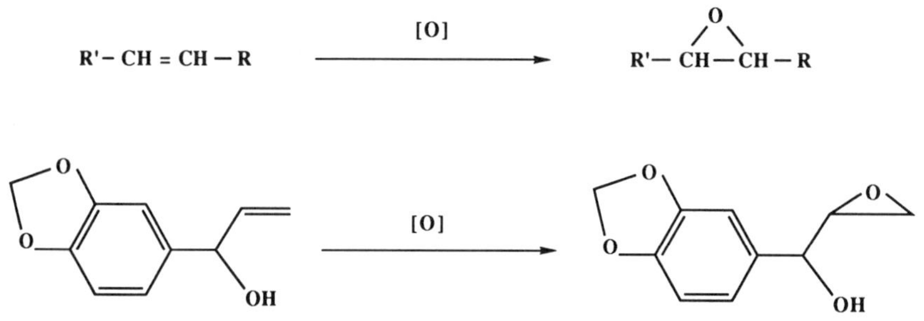

R'− CH = CH − R —[O]→ R'− CH(O)CH − R

1'-Hydroxysafrole —[O]→ 1'-Hydroxysafrole-2',3'-oxide

Figure 3.3 An oxidation process of Phase I reactions: epoxidation and a typical example.

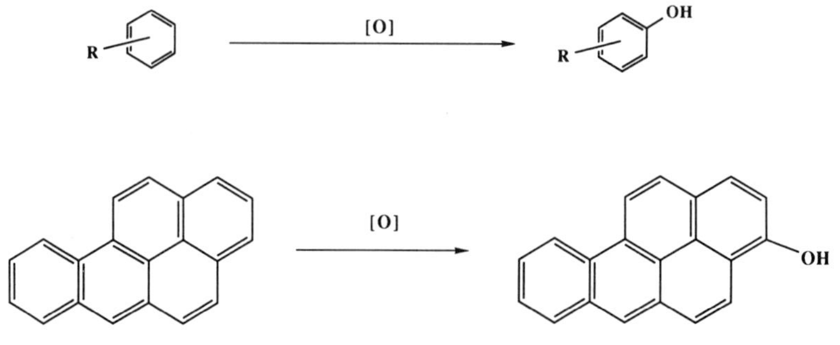

Benzo[a]pyrene —[O]→ 3-Hydroxybenzo[a]pyrene

Figure 3.4 An oxidation process of Phase I reactions: aromatic hydroxylation and a typical example.

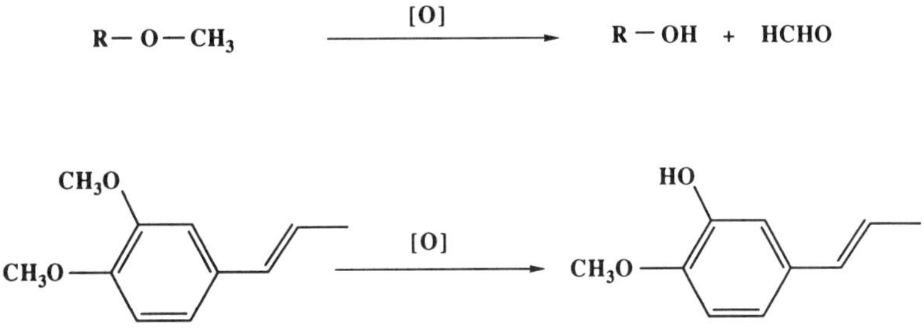

$$R-O-CH_3 \xrightarrow{[O]} R-OH + HCHO$$

3,4-Dimethoxy allylbenzene → 3-Hydroxy-4-methoxy allylbenzene

Figure 3.5 An oxidation process of Phase I reactions: *O*-dealkylation and a typical example.

$$R-S-CH_3 \xrightarrow{[O]} R-SH + HCHO$$

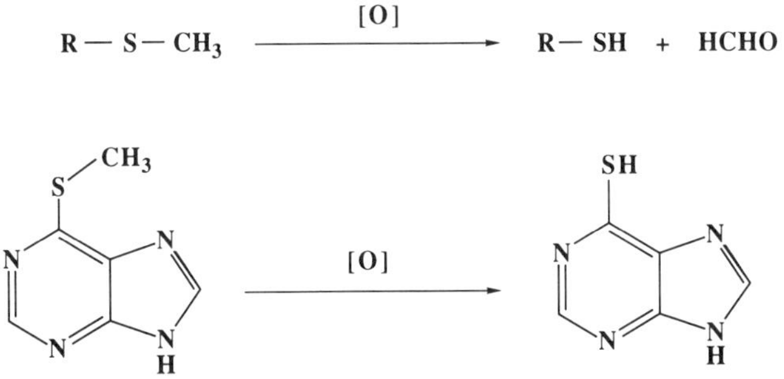

6-Methylthiopurine → 6-Mercaptopurine

Figure 3.6 An oxidation process of Phase I reactions: *S*-dealkylation and a typical example.

$$(RO)(R'O)P(=S)OR'' \xrightarrow{[O]} (RO)(R'O)P(=O)OR''$$

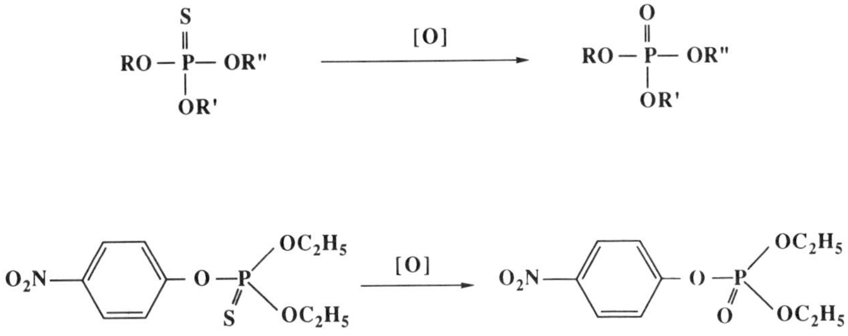

Parathion → Paraoxon

Figure 3.7 An oxidation process of Phase I reactions: desulfuration and a typical example.

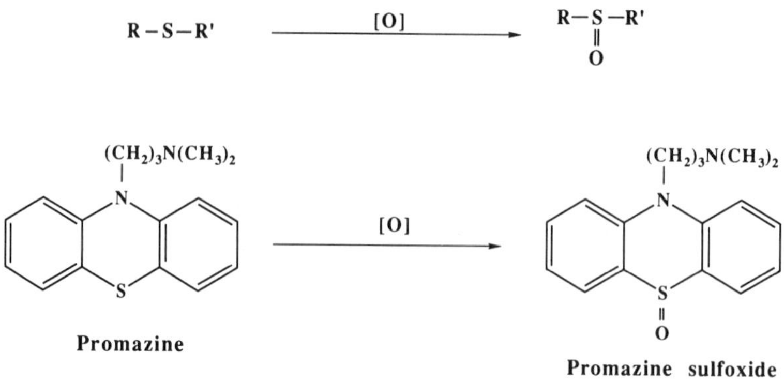

R–S–R' $\xrightarrow{[O]}$ R–S(=O)–R'

$(CH_2)_3N(CH_3)_2$ — Promazine $\xrightarrow{[O]}$ Promazine sulfoxide

Figure 3.8 An oxidation process of Phase I reactions: sulfoxidation and a typical example.

R–N(R')–H $\xrightarrow{[O]}$ R–N(OH)–R'

2-Acetylaminofluorene $\xrightarrow{[O]}$ N-Hydroxy-2-acetyl aminofluorene

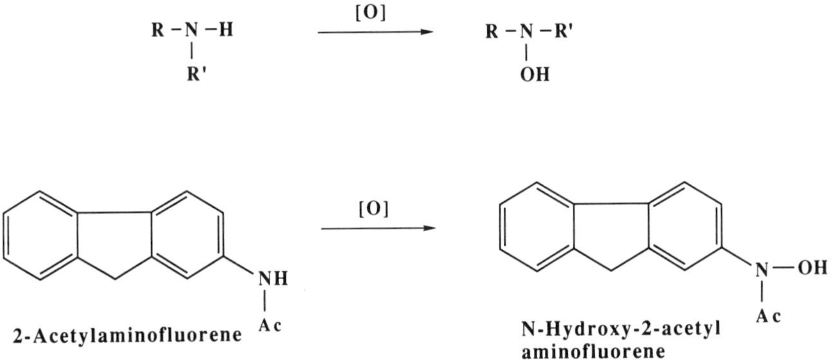

Figure 3.9 An oxidation process of Phase I reactions: *N*-oxidation and a typical example.

R–N(R')–CH_3 $\xrightarrow{[O]}$ R–NH–R'

Morphine $\xrightarrow{[O]}$ Normorphine

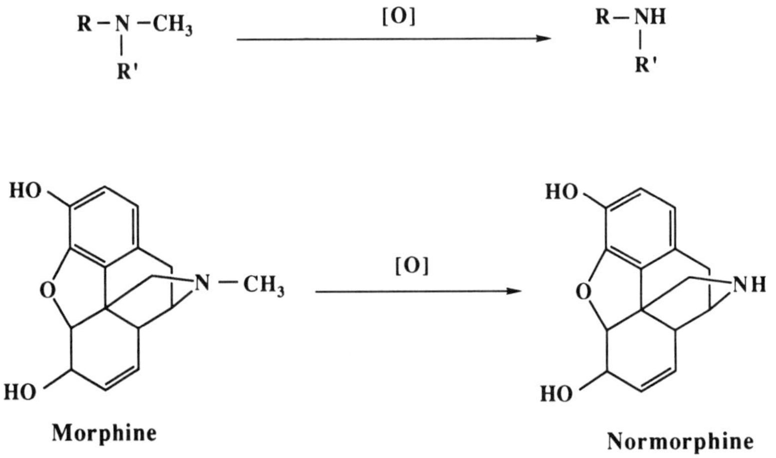

Figure 3.10 An oxidation process of Phase I reactions: *N*-dealkylation and a typical example.

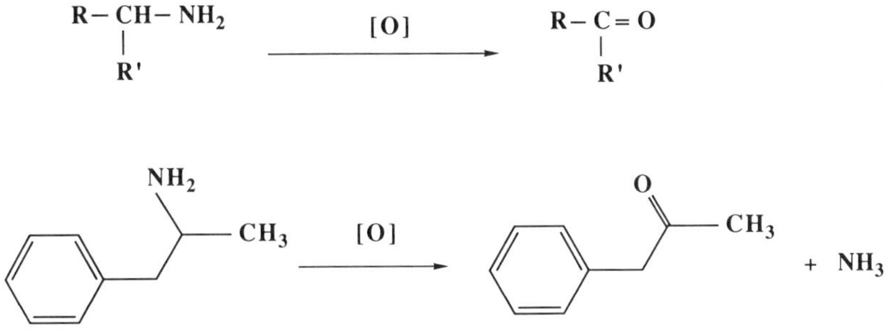

$$R-CH(R')-NH_2 \xrightarrow{[O]} R-C(R')=O$$

$$\text{Amphetamine} \xrightarrow{[O]} \text{Benzylmethylketone} + NH_3$$

Figure 3.11 An oxidation process of Phase I reactions: deamination and a typical example.

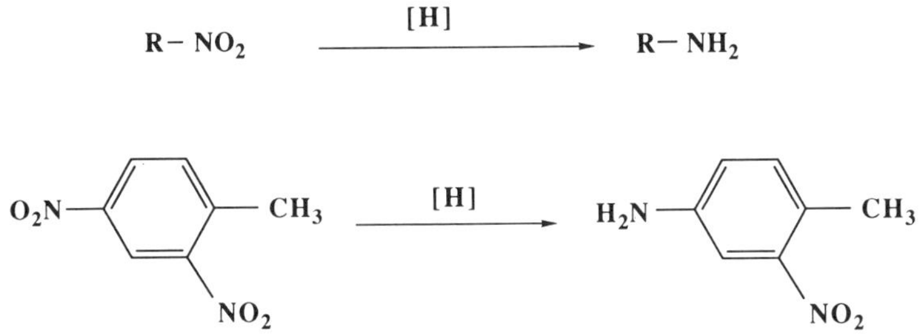

$$R-NO_2 \xrightarrow{[H]} R-NH_2$$

$$\text{2,4-Dinitrotoluene} \xrightarrow{[H]} \text{4-Amino-2-nitrotoluene}$$

Figure 3.12 A reduction process of Phase I reactions: nitro reduction and a typical example.

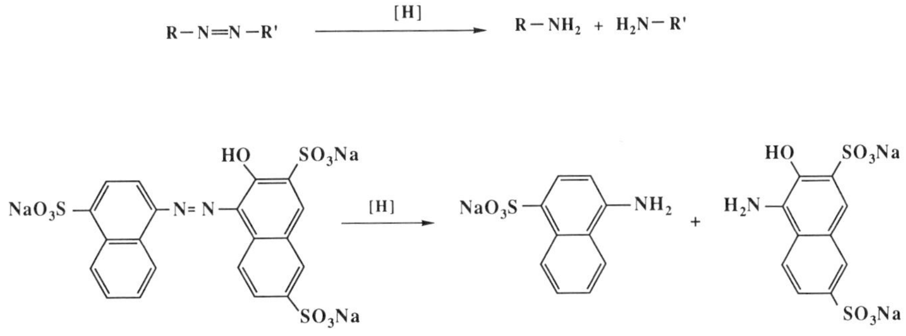

$$R-N{=}N-R' \xrightarrow{[H]} R-NH_2 + H_2N-R'$$

$$\text{FD \& C Red No. 2} \xrightarrow{[H]} \text{Naphthylamines}$$

Figure 3.13 A reduction process of Phase I reactions: azo reduction and a typical example.

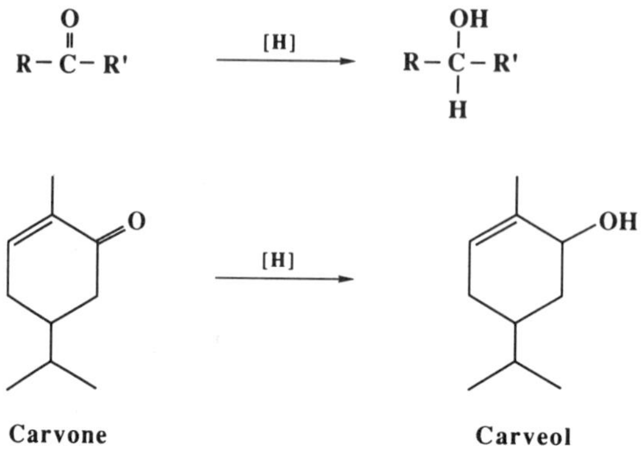

Carvone Carveol

Figure 3.14 A reduction process of Phase I reactions: carbonyl reduction and a typical example.

molecule that can be readily excreted, most often through the urine. Glucuronyl transferase, glutathione *S*-transferase (GST), and sulfotransferase are the most important enzymes in these Phase II processes. Glucuronyl transferase and sulfotransferase mediate the formal addition of glucuronic acid and sulfate, respectively, to various alcohols, carboxylic acids, sulfhydril, and amine compounds (Figure 3.3). GST mediates the formal addition of glutathione to various substances by displacement reactions. For example, GST mediates the addition of glutathione to chlorodinitrobenzene with the displacement of chloride. This class of displacement reactions is also important for the detoxification of certain epoxide derivatives yielding the corresponding thioalcohol. In this way, GST not only mediates the production of a more water-soluble substance but also participates in the direct detoxification of these epoxides.

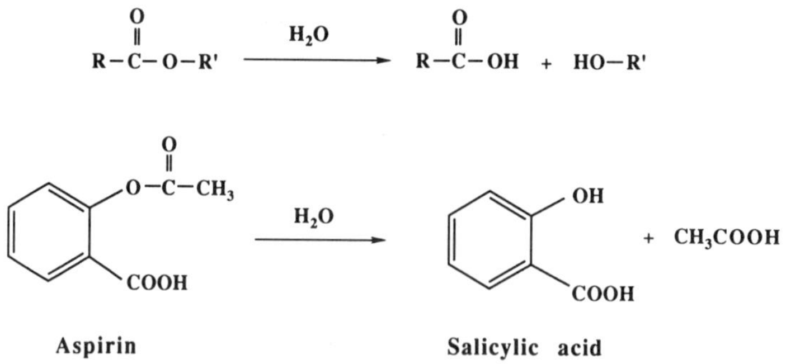

Aspirin Salicylic acid

Figure 3.15 A hydrolysis process of Phase I reactions: hydrolysis and a typical example.

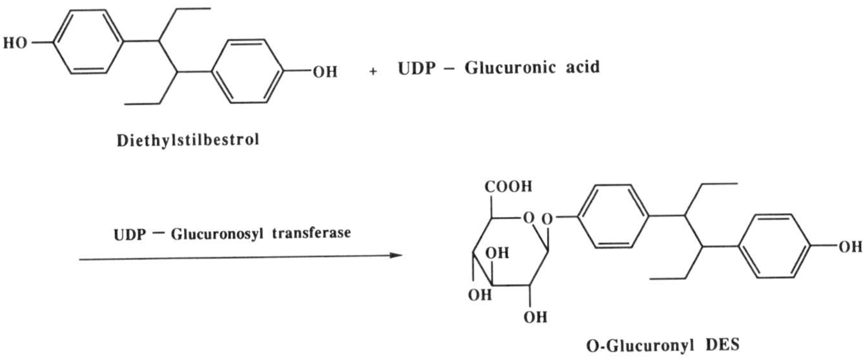

HO — OH + UDP – Glucuronic acid

Diethylstilbestrol

UDP — Glucuronosyl transferase

COOH O O OH OH OH OH

O-Glucuronyl DES

Figure 3.16 A conjugation process of Phase II reactions with glucuronic acid and a typical example.

The intracellular localization of the Phase II enzymes can influence the effectiveness of detoxification reactions. GST and sulfotransferase activities are present as soluble enzymes in the cytosol. GST is a major cytosolic enzyme in some tissues and comprises as much as 5% of the total soluble protein of the liver. In addition to its enzymatic function, a cytosolic GST known as ligandin is also important as a major binding protein. Thus, many xenobiotics are present in cells as non-covalently bound adducts with cytosolic GST. GST and glucuronyl transferase are also present in the nucleus and in membranes of the endoplasmic reticulum. Conjugation activity in these organelles can facilitate the rapid detoxification of activated xenobiotics produced by the cytochrome P450 systems also present there.

IV. The Effects of Diet on Biotransformation

Several characteristics of an organism can affect the toxicity of substances. Toxicity can be dependent on the species, sex, strain, circadian rhythms, and age of the test organism. These factors are genetically determined in

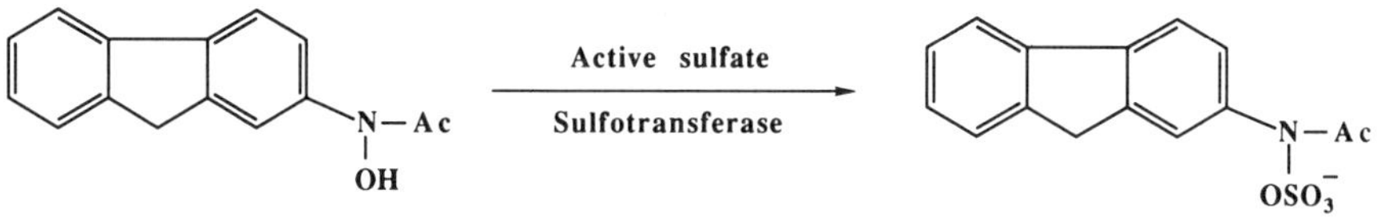

N—Ac OH

Active sulfate

Sulfotransferase

N—Ac OSO_3^-

Figure 3.17 A conjugation process of Phase II reactions with sulfate and a typical example.

the organism and may result from, for example, increased metabolic rates or incomplete development of a membrane or metabolic system. Factors external to the organism, such as diet, can also have marked effects on the toxicity of substances.

The effect of diet on toxicity may often be traced to alterations in the metabolic capacity of the organism. In theory, a deficiency in any of the several nutrients that are required for either Phase I or Phase II transformations could lead to decreased activity in these systems. However, variations in nutrient intake often lead to unexpected effects on toxicity.

In mice, short-term riboflavin deficiency results in an increase in levels of cytochrome P450 and an increase in the oxidation of certain substrates. Long-term riboflavin deficiency (7 weeks) is required to produce substantial decreases in P450 activity. Subsequent prolonged periods (10–15 days) of riboflavin supplementation are required before levels of components of the cytochrome P450 system approach normal values. Effects of riboflavin deficiency on NADPH–cytochrome P450 reductase are difficult to separate from the more general nutritional effect on the animal.

Vitamin E and vitamin C are two other nutrients that do not have an obvious direct role in Phase I oxidations. Vitamin E deficiency in rats decreases certain oxidative demethylation reactions. Vitamin E is a regulator of heme synthesis and heme is an essential component of cytochrome P450. Vitamin C deficiency results in the decreased metabolism of many substances with a decrease in cytochrome P450 and NADPH–cytochrome P450 reductase. Although the mechanism of this effect is not understood, ascorbic acid deficiency appears to decrease the stability of the metabolic system. Hepatic microsomal cytochrome P450 isolated from ascorbic acid-deficient animals is less stable to sonication, dialysis, or treatment with iron chelators compared to cytochrome P450 from animals fed ascorbic acid-supplemented diets.

Protein deficiency affects metabolism of many substances and increases or decreases toxicity depending on the specific compound. Protein deficiency leads to a reduction in levels of NADPH–cytochrome P450 reductase and of certain cytochrome P450 isoenzymes. Protein supplementation of deficient diets results in the restoration of metabolic rates for certain substrates but not for others. The reason for these specific effects of protein deficiency on various enzyme systems in the microsomal metabolic apparatus is not understood.

The effects of dietary fat on the microsomal metabolic apparatus depend on the type of fat and the quantity and the type of substance being metabolized. For example, increased levels of saturated fatty acids in the diet produce increased levels of aniline oxidation with no increase in hexobarbital oxidation, but supplementation with unsaturated fats results in increased metabolic rates for several substances with an attendant increase in concentration of cytochrome P450 and decreased glucose-6-phosphate dehydrogenase activity.

Modification of intake of certain minerals also affects rates of metabolism of various substances in laboratory animals. For example, iron deficiency leads to a marked stimulation in hepatic metabolism of many substances. However, iron deficiency apparently has little effect on the levels of cytochrome P450 or cytochrome P450 reductase in liver tissues. Cytochrome P450 activity in the small intestine of rats is highly sensitive to dietary iron. Deficiency of this metal produces a rapid drop in the activities of several P450-associated enzymes.

Magnesium deficiency causes a marked decrease in metabolism of xenobiotics in the liver with lower levels of hepatic cytochrome P450 and cytochrome P450 reductase. Decreased levels of these essential components may account at least in part for the lower metabolic rate of xenobiotics in the livers of malnourished individuals. Explanations for the effects of dietary minerals on liver-mediated metabolism of xenobiotics await further studies.

V. Metabolic Induction

The activity or levels of certain components of the hepatic metabolic apparatus of many organisms are increased by exposure to a large variety of drugs, carcinogens, and other foreign compounds. Induction of the hepatic oxidase system is directly attributable to an increase in the amount of cytochrome P450 and other microsomal proteins within the cell. The process requires an increase in RNA synthesis and a subsequent increase in protein synthesis.

Treatment of animals with different inducers, such as 3-methylcholanthrene and phenobarbital, results in differential effects on the rate of hydroxylation of various compounds. For example, 3-methylcholanthrene and similar inducers tend to increase the rate of hydroxylation of polycyclic aromatic hydrocarbons and induce the formation of a slightly different cytochrome (now called CYP1A1), which has an absorption maximum at 448 nm instead of 450 nm. In contrast, phenobarbital treatment results in an increase of CYP2B1 and corresponding increases in rates of metabolism of hexobarbital and aminopyrine.

The list of enzyme-inducing agents has grown to include several classes of foreign compounds that are widespread in the environment. Among them are polycyclic aromatic hydrocarbons, halogenated hydrocarbons, nicotine and other alkaloids, food additives used as antioxidants, coloring agents, and naturally occurring components in many foods. While these classifications cover a broad spectrum of compounds, two primary features common to these agents are

1. they are lipid soluble and thus become localized within the smooth endoplasmic reticulum, and
2. they are substrates of, or become bound to, cytochrome P450 or other microsomal enzymes.

One group of foods which induces microsomal enzyme activity is the cruciferous vegetables including Brussels sprouts, cabbage, broccoli, and cauliflower. Dietary cruciferous vegetables produce more than a 100-fold increase in the CYP1A enzymes in the small intestine of rats.

Certain indoles (Figure 3.18) that are components of many cruciferous vegetables have significant inducing effects on microsomal enzymes. When administered to rats as single purified substances, some of these indoles increase CYP1A1 activity greater than 200-fold in the intestine and 30- to 40-fold in the liver. These indoles account for the majority of the inducing effects of the vegetables. Indole-3-carbinol is not an active inducing agent by itself but is converted to active substances when it contacts aqueous acid either *in vitro* or *in vivo* in the stomach. One highly active product of indole-3-carbinol and possibly other dietary indoles is ICZ (indolo[3,2-*b*]carbozole). The biological effects of ICZ and other products of indole-3-carbinol are currently under study.

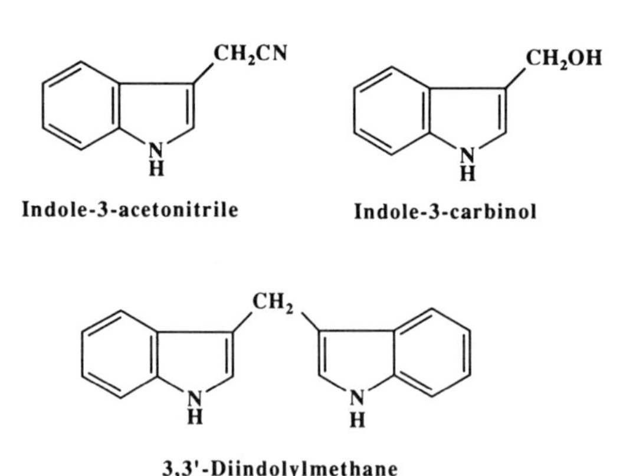

Figure 3.18 Structures of indole derivatives.

Food-borne substances can affect activities of other drug-metabolizing enzymes. For example, activities of epoxide hydrolase in rat liver are increased to 2- to 4-fold by treatment with substances such as phenobarbital, 3-methylcholanthrene, and BHA. An increase in UDP–glucuronyl transferase activity is also seen when animals are exposed to a number of these substances. GST activity is also increased as a result of induction by natural substances (such as goitrin) from cruciferous vegetables.

In general, it is not possible to predict, on the basis of data currently available, the overall effect of enzyme-inducing agents on the toxicity of xenobiotics. Inducing agents generally affect several enzymes in the metabolic system with a considerably more complicated metabolic result than might be expected from a change in the activity of a single enzyme. For example, increased levels of cytochrome P450-mediated oxidation of a polycyclic aromatic hydrocarbon should result in increased levels of activated substances such as epoxides, which, in turn, should yield increased levels of toxicity. However, concomitant induction of one of the detoxification and conjugation systems such as GST and glucuronyl transferases along with the cytochrome P450 system can lead to an overall increased rate of metabolism and excretion of the substance, thereby rendering the substance less toxic. Based on the available experimental evidence, it appears that most substances that tend to increase levels of microsomal oxidation lead to an overall decrease in toxicity of many substances. For example, administration of the indoles previously mentioned as components of certain cruciferous vegetables inhibits benzo[*a*]pyrene-induced neoplasia in the forestomach of mice and inhibits 7,12-dimethylbenzo[*a*]anthracene-induced mammary tumor formation in rats.

Even in this brief discussion it becomes apparent that biotransformation is an important and complex process. Individual variation in susceptibility to toxic agents may be related to genetic or environmentally induced variations in biotransformation. As our understanding of biotransformation in humans grows, it may be possible to explain and predict individual differences in susceptibility to toxic agents.

Suggestions for Further Reading

1. Albert, A. (1987). "Xenobiosis: Foods, Drugs, and Poisons in the Human Body." Chapman and Hall, New York.
2. Anders, M. W. (ed.) (1985). Bioactivation of foreign compounds. *In* "Biochemical Pharmacology and Toxicology." Academic Press, Orlando.
3. Anderson, K. E., Pantuck, E. J., Conney, A. H., and Kappas, A. (1985). Nutrient regulation of chemical metabolism in humans. *Fed. Proc.* **44,** 130.

4. Boyd, E. M. (1972). "Protein Deficiency and Pesticide Toxicity." Charles C. Thomas, Springfield.
5. Caldwell, J., and Paulson, G. D. (1964). "Foreign Compound Metabolism." Taylor & Francis, Philadelphia.
6. Caldwell, J., and Jakoby, W. B. (eds.) (1983). Biological basis of detoxication. *In* "Biochemical Pharmacology and Toxicology." Academic Press, New York.
7. Committee on Diet, Nutrition, and Cancer, NRC. (1982). "Diet, Nutrition, and Cancer." National Academy Press, Washington, D.C.
8. Finley, J. W., and Schwasss, D. E. (eds.) (1985). "Xenobiotic Metabolism: Nutritional Effects." ACS symposium series 277, American Chemical Society, Washington, D.C..
9. Gram, T. E. (ed.) (1980). "Extrahepatic Metabolism of Drugs and Other Foreign Compounds." SP Medical and Scientific Books, New York.
10. Hathcock, J. N., and Coon, J. (eds.) (1978). "Nutrition and Drug Interrelations." Academic Press, New York.
11. Hawkins, D. R. (1988). "Biotransformations: A Survey of the Biotransformations of Drugs and Chemicals in Animals." Royal Society of Chemistry, London.
12. Jakoby, W. B., Bend, J. R., and Caldwell, J. (eds.) (1982). Metabolic basis of detoxication: Metabolism of functional groups. *In* "Biochemical Pharmacology and Toxicology." Academic Press, New York.
13. Miyamoto, J., Kaneko, H., Hutson, D. H., Esser, H. O., Gorbach, S., and Dorn, E. (1988). "Pesticide Metabolism: Extrapolation from Animals to Man." Blackwell Scientific, Boston.
14. Paulson, G. D., Menn, J. J., Caldwell, J., and Hutson, D. H. (eds.) (1986). "Xenobiotic Conjugation Chemistry." ACS symposium series 299, American Chemical Society, Washington, D. C.
15. Turnbull, J. D., and Omaye, S. T. (1980). Synthesis of cytochrome-P450 heme in ascorbic acid-deficient guinea pigs. *Biochem. Pharmacol.* **29,** 1255.
16. Klaassen, C. D., Amdur, M. O., and Doull, J. (1986). The basic science of poisons. *In* "Toxicology" (L. J. Casarett and J. Doull, eds), 3rd Ed. Macmillan, New York.
17. Loomis, T. A. (1978). "Essentials of Toxicology," 3rd Ed. Lea and Febiger, Philadelphia.

CHAPTER 4

Natural Toxins in Animal Foodstuffs

Since humans first evolved, the search for food has been one of their primary activities. It is hypothesized that people were originally vegetarians and gradually adapted foods from animal sources. In particular, mastery of the use of fire about 75,000 years ago dramatically increased the variety of foods. Over time, people learned that heat treatment detoxified certain poisonous foods. As more and better ways of processing foodstuffs have been learned, the variety of foods available for human consumption has increased.

I. Toxins Occurring in Animal Liver

The animal liver, a large glandular organ, is a nutritious protein-rich food in which important enzymes are concentrated. Beef, calf, pork, and lamb livers are commonly sold in Western markets.

A. Bile Acids

Some livers—bear, beef, sheep, goat, and rabbit—produce toxic acids called bile acid. In dried bear liver, the bile acid acts as a suppressant (both as a tranquilizer and as a pain killer) on the central nervous system. The Chinese and Japanese discovered this long ago and used dried bear liver as one of their folk medicines over the centuries. Bile acids are cholic acid, deoxycholic acid, and taurocholic acid, and are shown in decreasing order of toxicity in Figure 4.1.

The livers commonly eaten as food in the Western World do not contain sufficient quantities of bile acids to produce toxic effects. It is, however, necessary to be aware that not only bear liver but also most other animal livers contain toxic acids that may be poisonous when consumed in large quantities. In addition, animal studies have shown that bile acids can promote tumor formation in the bowel.

B. Vitamin A

Vitamin A is necessary for normal growth and vision in animals. A deficiency of vitamin A can lead to night blindness, failure of normal bone growth in the young, and diseases of the membranes of the nose, throat, and eyes. Vitamin A is a fat-soluble, light yellow substance that crystallizes as needles (MP 63°C). β-Carotene, which breaks down into two molecules of vitamin A in the intestinal mucosa (Figure 4.2), is manufactured in plants and stored in the liver and fat of animals as the palmitate ester.

Generally, vitamin A is toxic to humans at the level of 2–5 million IU (International Unit is a standardized measure of a vitamin's biological activity). One IU corresponds to 0.3 mg of pure crystalline vitamin A. Polar bear liver is very rich in vitamin A and at least one case of acute intoxication due to the consumption of the vitamin A-rich liver was reported among Arctic explorers and their dogs. The ingestion of the liver of polar bears produced a painful swelling under the skin. In other reported instances, ingestion of polar bear livers caused joint pain and irritation, dry lips, lip bleeding, and ultimately death. There is also a report that a fisherman who ingested nearly 30 million IU of vitamin A in halibut liver, which contains up to 100,000 IU/g of vitamin A, complained of severe headache centered in the forehead and eyes, dizziness, drowsiness, nausea, and vomiting followed by redness and erythematous swelling and peeling of the skin.

In Table 4.1 the vitamin A content in the livers of various animals is shown. Ingestion of approximately 111 to 278 g of polar bear liver causes acute vitamin A toxicity. Chronic vitamin A toxicity is induced by 1000 mg (approximately 3000 IU)/kg body weight/day. Values vary from source to source but this is the value that is commonly recognized.

It is difficult to define the toxicity of excessive levels of essential nutrients because any food can cause a toxic reaction if it is ingested in excessive amounts. Vitamin A, therefore, is not classified as a toxic material even though excessive consumption results in a toxic response.

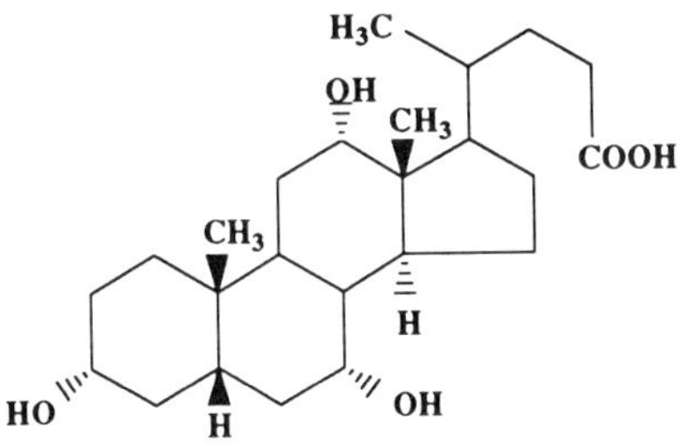

Cholic acid

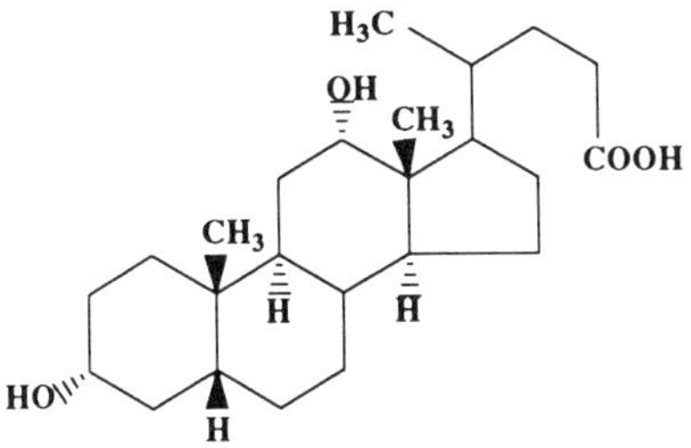

Deoxycholic acid

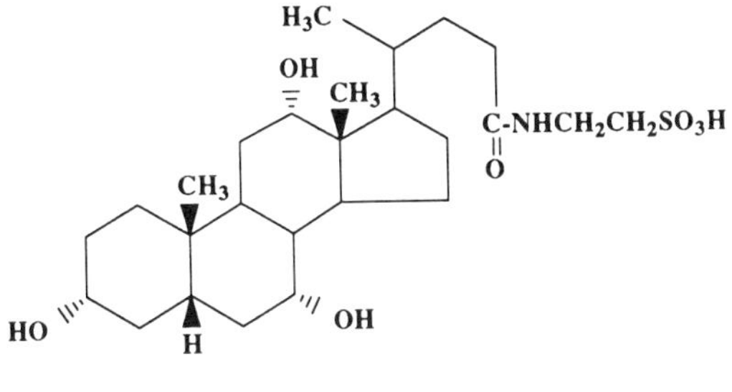

Taurocholic acid

Figure 4.1 Structures of bile acids.

II. Toxins Occurring in Marine Animals

Americans currently consume approximately 13 lb of fish per capita per year, a figure which represents less than 10% of their meat consumption; this indicates that seafood is not an important part of the diet of most

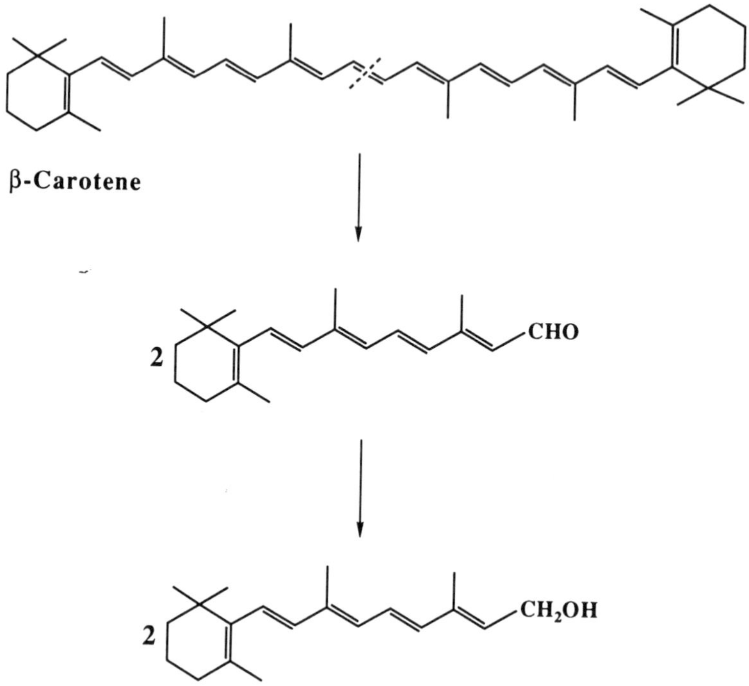

β-Carotene

CHO

2

CH_2OH

2

Vitamin A

Figure 4.2 Formation of vitamin A from β-carotene.

people in the United States. However, in parts of the world such as Southeast Asia and southern Europe, fish is one of the most important sources of protein.

Fish tissue, which is more perishable than animal tissue, is very susceptible to microorganism invasion. This is why freshly caught fish stored at a moderate temperature of 60°F will remain unspoiled for only 1 day

TABLE 4.1
Animals Containing High Levels of Vitamin A in Liver

Animal	Content (IU/100 g fresh)
Polar bear	1.8 million
Seal	1.3 million
Sheep or cattle	4000–45,000
(Butter)	2400–4000

or less. Table 4.2 shows the approximate number of days certain fish stored at certain temperatures can be expected to remain in an unspoiled condition.

Food poisoning not involving microorganism action is mostly caused by marine animals; instances of poison occurring in land animals are extremely rare. Some examples of poisonous marine animals with the types of poison they contain are shown in Table 4.3.

A. Scombroid Poisoning

The majority of seafood poisoning cases are attributed to bacterial decomposition of improperly stored fish. Because of the widespread consumption of *Scombroidea* species (which include mackerel, tuna, bluefish, and skipjack), seafood poisoning has become associated with these species and is therefore called scombroid poisoning. However, many non-scombroid species have been implicated in outbreaks, including mahi-mahi, sardines, anchovies, and herring.

Symptoms of scombroid poisoning may begin to appear 2 hr after ingestion of contaminated fish, and the poisoning usually runs its course within 16 hr. There are generally no lasting ill effects and fatalities are very rare. The gastrointestinal tract is affected in most (but not all) cases, giving rise to pain, nausea, vomiting, and diarrhea. These symptoms are often accompanied by neurological and cutaneous symptoms such as headache, tingling, flushing, or urticaria.

These symptoms resemble allergic reactions caused by histidine. Therefore, scombroid poisoning has been attributed to the histamine produced by bacterial decarboxylation of the amino acid histidine in fish. This reaction is illustrated in Figure 4.3. Histamine can reach concentrations of up to 5 mg/g in fish without the development of off-flavors that would cause it to be rejected. In most cases, analysis of fish samples

TABLE 4.2
Periods of Time for Certain Kinds of Fish to Remain in an Unspoiled Condition

Fish products	At 32°F	At 60°F
Fresh cod	14 days	1 day
Fresh salmon	12 days	1 day
Salted herring	1 year	3–4 months
Dried salted cod	1 year	4–6 months

TABLE 4.3
Type of Poison Found in Various Marine Animals

Marine animal	Type of poison
Sea anemone, jellyfish, octopus	Protein
Abalones	Pyropheophorbide *a*
Shellfishes, crabs	Saxitoxin
Pufferfish (blowfish or fugu), California newt	Tetrodotoxin
Snappers, barracudas, seabasses, sharks, eels, parrotfish	Ciguatoxin

involved in scombroid poisoning shows high histidine levels. However, pure histamine has relatively low oral toxicity in humans. Oral ingestion of up to 180 mg leads to no observable effects, while intravenous administration of less than 10 mg produces detectable cardiovascular effects. It appears that other substances in the fish such as putrescine and cadaverine trigger the toxicity of histamine.

B. Saxitoxin

One of the most serious threats to public health posed by fish is known as paralytic shellfish poisoning (PSP). This is associated with the phenomenon of "red tides" or blooms, which occur when certain species of algae, the dinoflagellates, undergo rapid growth, resulting in up to one million of these organisms per milliliter of seawater. Visible blooms can appear at concentrations of roughly 20,000 organisms/ml and may vary in color according to the species involved. However, toxicity can develop in the absence of observable color. A few species of dinoflagellates, in particular *Gonylaux* sp., produce a toxin that accumulates in shellfish such as clams or mussels feeding on these algae. It appears that the toxin has no ill effects on the shellfish, but small amounts are highly toxic to humans and there is no known antidote. The toxin cannot be removed by washing and is unaffected by heat. Blooms are short-lived, lasting 2 to 3 weeks,

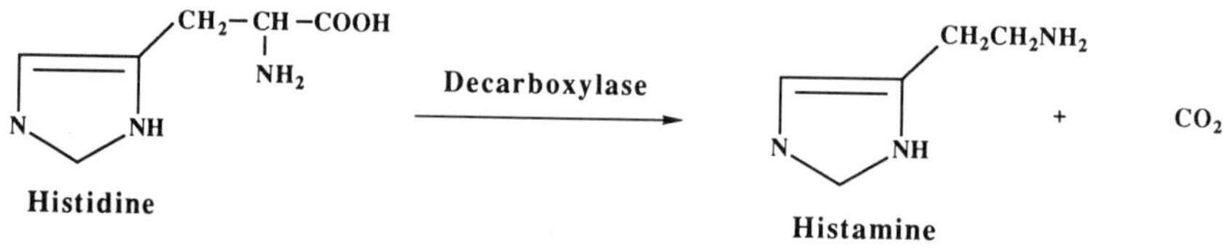

Histidine ($CH_2-CH(NH_2)-COOH$ on imidazole ring) —Decarboxylase→ Histamine ($CH_2CH_2NH_2$ on imidazole ring) + CO_2

Figure 4.3 Bacterial decarboxylation of the amino acid histidine in fish.

and most shellfish break down or excrete the toxin within 3 weeks after ingestion stops. Thus, affected shellfish are only occasionally toxic. However, in certain species of clams, the toxin is distributed throughout the organism, which can then remain toxic for months.

PSP has occurred throughout the world, generally in regions 30 degrees or higher in latitude. It is common in coastal waters of the North Sea in Europe, North America, Japan, and South Africa. While the phenomenon of PSP had been recognized for centuries in these areas, it was not until 1937 that the association with dinoflagellates was established.

In early work on PSP, the poison was identified by a bioassay in mice. An extract of the shellfish was serially diluted and injected intraperitoneally. The level of dilution that produced death within 15 min came to be defined as one "mouse unit" of toxin. After the pure toxin (saxitoxin) was isolated, it was found that one MU was equal to 0.18 μg or a dose of 9 $\mu g/kg$ for a 20-g mouse. In laboratory animals, oral toxicity is roughly one-tenth that of an IP injection. The estimated minimum lethal dose in humans is 4 mg or less and a dose of 1 mg is estimated to cause mild intoxication.

Of all toxic compounds from marine organisms, saxitoxin (Figure 4.4) has been of considerable importance due to its mammalian toxicity. Problems associated with saxitoxin are not new. The red color of the saxitoxin-infested seawater caused by the sudden bloom of microalgae with protozoans, bacteria, and other microorganisms was well known by the West Coast Indians of North America. They recognized the red tides which preceded the intake of saxitoxin-infected mussels and stationed guards to note the first signs of the colored water in order to prevent the taking of mussels until the color returned to normal. Although red tide

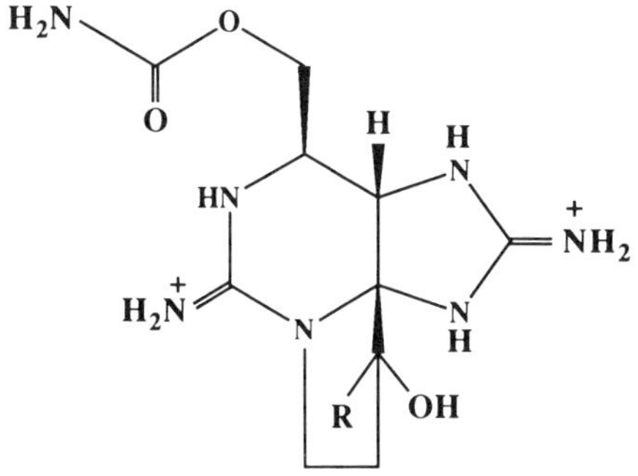

H_2N O O H H N HN $\overset{+}{N}H_2$ $H_2\overset{+}{N}$ N N H R OH

Figure 4.4 Structure of saxitoxin.

and associated saxitoxin poisoning have occurred throughout the world, it has been studied most intensively in North America where major problems have been identified.

1. Occurrence in Crabs

There are more than 20 different species of crabs eaten around the world and all contain greater or lesser quantities of toxic materials. It is still not clear how these crabs produce poisonous materials, but the sand crab, *Emerita analoga,* becomes poisonous when living in an area affected by the red tide which carries poisonous algae (*Gonyaulax* spp.). Three species of *Santhidae—Zosiums aeneus, Platypodia granulosa, Atergatis floridus*—are known to be poisonous and all are found in the South Pacific. Table 4.4 shows the poison content in each part of the *Z. aeneus.*

2. Occurrence in Shellfishes

There are about 28 species of shellfish in the world that are used for food. Most kinds of shellfish contain somewhat toxic materials and only those shellfish found in the Mediterranean Sea and the Red Sea are known not to be poisonous. The shellfish collected in the Gulf of Mexico are also less poisonous than those indigenous to other areas. Generally, the shellfish themselves do not produce toxic materials but rather become poisonous through their association with algae. *Gonyaulax catenella, Gonyaulax acatnell, Gonyaulax tamarensis, Pyrimidium phoenus, Exuviaella mariaele-*

TABLE 4.4
Distribution of Toxin in the Body of Crab (*Z. aneneus*)

Part of the body	Toxicity (MU/g)
Appendages	
Exoskeleton of chela	2000
Muscle of chela	6000
Exoskeleton of walking legs	2000
Muscle of walking legs	3500
Cephalothorax	
Exoskeleton	2000
Muscle	40
Viscera	1300
Endophragm	80
Gill	25

bovriae, and *Gymnodinium breve* have been directly involved in causing shellfish to become poisonous enough to cause food poisoning in humans. On the West Coast, the dinoflagellate *Gonyaulax catenella* infects the mollusks *Mytilus californianus* (common mussel) and *Saxidonus giganteus* (Alaskan butter clam). *Gonyaulax tamarensis* is the East Coast equivalent, infecting the *Mytilus edulis* (mussel), *Mya arenaria* (clam), and *Plocopecten magellanicus* (scallop). In Europe and Japan, unknown algae infect *M. edulis* and *Carassostrea gigas* (oyster), respectively. *Gonyaulax* sp. have also been implicated in saxitoxin poisoning from mussels, clams, oysters, cockles, and scallops in the Indo-Pacific.

3. Mode of Action and Toxicities

Pure saxitoxin was isolated from California mussels and Alaska butter clams in 1954. Symptoms of a fatal toxic reaction from saxitoxin poisoning are numbness of lips, hands, and feet 15 min to 2–3 hr after ingestion of the poisoned shellfish. This is followed by difficulty in walking, vomiting, coma, and death.

The LD_{50} of saxitoxin in mice (IP injection) is 10 μg/kg. Seven related saxitoxin-like compounds have been isolated from dinoflagellates and from mollusks, and recent work has shown that shellfish tissues are capable of biotransformations of these quaternary ammonium salts.

The toxicity of saxitoxin is expressed in mouse units (MU); that is, the amount of toxin that kills a mouse (20 g body weight Swiss Webster mouse) in 15 min. The curve shown in Figure 4.5 indicates the dose-related death time on mice for *Z. aeneus* crab toxin.

Programs like the Mussel Watch Program in California provide the best solution to the problem of saxitoxin poisoning. Good prevention programs include the monitoring of deaths of mullusk predators and signs of red tides and—most importantly—stressing "if in doubt, throw it out" to shellfish consumers.

By 1976 some 1600 known cases of PSP had been reported in Spain, Germany, Japan, Malaysia, Canada, and the United States. In addition to causing health problems, PSP outbreaks also damage shellfish industries. In 1972, local fishermen in New England lost an estimated one million dollars due to PSP contamination. Recently, International Shellfish Industries of Moss Landing, California was forced into closure when it had to cancel all shipping to overseas markets. Their entire stock of seed oysters had been contaminated.

In the United States, the Federal government has been trying to protect people from paralytic shellfish poisoning since 1925. In 1951, the FDA (Food and Drug Administration) issued regulations limiting the PSP

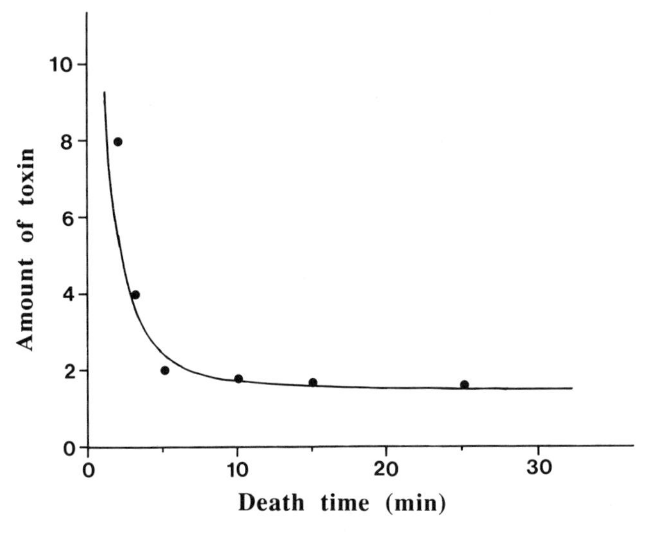

Figure 4.5 The dose–death time curve for a toxin in mice.

content of toxin in frozen or canned shellfish to 400 MU/100 g. Since 1958, the maximum allowable amount of saxitoxin in seafood products has been 80 μg/100 g. If the edible parts of shellfish in a culturing area contain more than 80 μg/100 g, commercial fishing is prohibited.

C. Tetramine

Tetramine is the major component of the salivary poison of the marine gastropods of the family Buccinidae (whelk, sea snail). The salivary gland of *Neptunea arthritica* contains 7 to 9 mg tetramine/g of gland. The Swedish species *Neptunea antiqua* contains as much as 20 to 30 mg/g of gland. Symptoms of tetramine poisoning are headache localized in the back of the head, dizziness, loss of balance, eye pain, vomiting, and hives. Recovery usually occurs within several hours.

Toxicity tests of salivary poison and of authentic tetramine for fish (*Cyprinus caprpio*) are carried out by submuscular injection, or by per os administration using a polyethlene catheter. After either injection or administration, the following symptoms are observed: gradual loss of balance, inversion of the abdomen, delayed respiration rate, clinical convulsion, and, finally, death.

D. *Pyropheophorbide* a

Abalone contains a toxic material called pyropheophorbide *a* (Figure 4.6) in its internal organs. It is a derivative of chlorophyll which may come from seaweed, but it is not clear why it accumulates in the liver of abalones only during the spring season. Because pyropheophorbide *a* is photoactive, it causes a toxic reaction if an individual eats the organs containing this compound (people in northern part of Japan eat them salted) and then is exposed to sunlight. Photosensitizers in the body promote the production of amine compounds from histidine, tryptophan, and tyrosine that cause inflammation and toxic reactions. The general symptom of photosensitized pyropheophorbide *a* poisoning is the appearance of red edema on face and hands; however, this toxin does not cause death.

E. *Tetrodotoxin*

Tetrodotoxin, also known as puffer or fugu poison, is associated primarily with the reproductive organs of fish. This toxin is found in many species of puffer fish (*Sphaeroides*), ocean sunfish, and porcupine fish. It is also

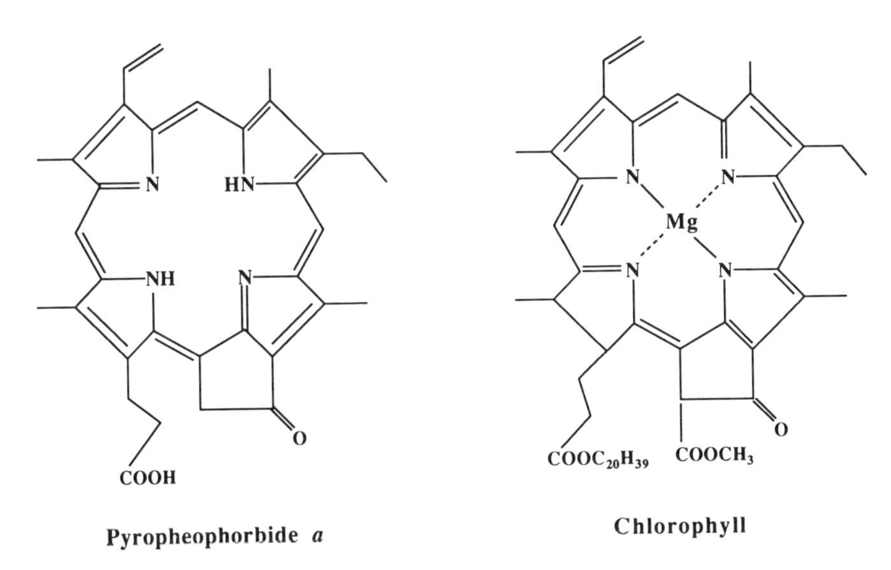

Figure 4.6 Structure of pyropheophorbide *a* and chlorophyll.

produced by certain amphibians in South America and Africa and has been collected from them for use as arrow poison. Most cases of human food poisoning by tetrodotoxin involve the puffer fish. These are considered a delicacy in Japan, at least in part because of the risks of eating puffer from which the poison has not been removed.

Certain species of puffer fish, particularly Fugu rubripes, are very popular in international cuisine; in Japan, statistics show that over 50 people are poisoned by fugu puffer fish annually. Deaths caused by fugu poisoning constitute 60–70% of the total deaths by food poisoning in Japan. Over 1000 cases of fugu poisoning have been reported in every decade during the last 100 years in Japan. The fatality rate has decreased from 87 to 32% during the last 100 years. The most enjoyable aspects of eating puffer fish, the slight numbness of the lips and tongue and sensation of warmth, are clear signs of mild tetrodotoxin intoxication.

1. Occurrence

No other naturally occurring animal toxins have received as much attention as tetrodotoxin. Toxicity of puffer fish was described as early as the second century in China. Later it was found that the California newt contained a toxin that was identical to tetrodotoxin.

In most tetrodotoxic species, the highest concentrations of the toxin are found in the ovaries, roe, and liver with lesser amounts in the skin and intestines. Small amounts can be found in the muscles and blood. Concentrations are generally higher in females and the occurrence and level of toxin are related to the spawning cycle of each species. Levels peak in winter, when connoisseurs consider the flavor of the fish to be best. About 80 of the puffer fish species *Tetraodoniformes* are known to contain or are suspected of containing tetrodotoxin. The toxin is present in the ovaries and eggs of the female and the content varies with the season (Figure 4.7). Since the quantity of tetrodotoxin in the muscle of the fish is very low, poisoning most frequently results from contamination of the edible parts of the fish with the ovaries or liver, or from direct ingestion of these internal organs.

2. Mode of Toxic Action and Toxicities

The symptoms of tetrodotoxin intoxication generally appear within 30–60 min (occasionally even earlier) and the typical progress of intoxication by tetrodotoxin occurs in four stages:

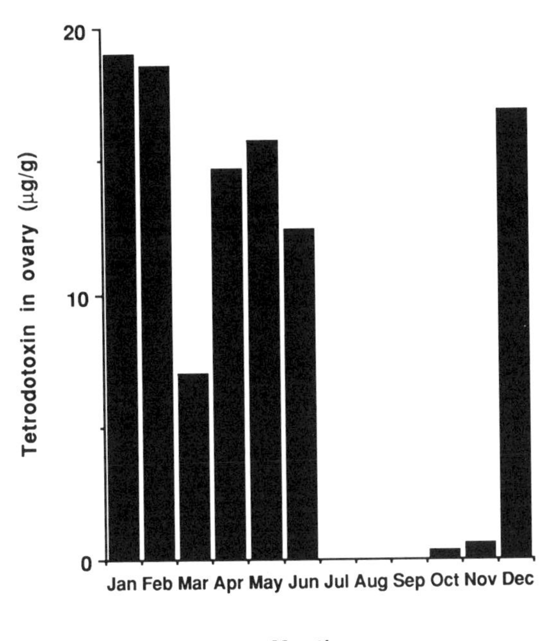

Figure 4.7 The concentrations of toxin present in the ovaries and eggs of the female puffer fish during different months.

1. Numbness of the lips, tongue, and often of fingers develops; nausea, vomiting, and anxiety follow.
2. Numbness becomes more marked; there is muscular paralysis of extremities without loss of tendon reflexes.
3. Ataxia (lack of muscular coordination) become more severe; paralysis develops. Consciousness is present, but speaking is difficult because of paralysis.
4. Consciousness is lost; death results from respiratory paralysis.

The prognosis for recovery from tetrodotoxin poisoning is unfavorable if the symptoms develop rapidly. If vomiting is severe, or if the symptoms are in the third and fourth stage, there is no antidote. Currently, the best treatment for tetrodotoxin poisoning is to remove the poison from the gastrointestinal tract and to apply artificial respiration.

Because tetrodotoxin is not antigenic, there is no antiserum. The fatal oral dose for humans is about 1–2 mg of crystalline tetrodotoxin, which is equivalent to approximately 1 g of the ovary from a highly toxic species captured during the winter; usually more than 10 g of roe is needed to produce fatal poisoning. Most cases of tetrodotoxin poisoning occur in Japan because of the presence of the highly toxic puffer fish and the common use of these fish as food.

The LD_{50} of tetrodotoxin to mice (intraperitoneally injection) is 10 μg/kg, which is almost the same as that of saxitoxin. However, tetrodotoxin when taken orally is absorbed much better than that of saxitoxin and is absorbed even through oral mucous membranes. When the tetrodotoxin is absorbed it blocks the flow of sodium ions into neurons and disrupts the transmission of nerve impulses.

3. Chemistry of Tetrodotoxin

In 1909, a crude sample of the principal fugu poison (0.2%) was isolated and named tetrodotoxin. Additional chemical studies on tetrodotoxin have been conducted since then and many researchers have tried to elucidate its very complex structure. X-ray analyses of certain tetrodotoxin derivatives have finally enabled researchers to understand its structure (Figure 4.8) and to subsequently develop the chemical synthesis of tetrodotoxin.

Tetrodotoxin is an amino perhydroquinazoline compound with a molecular formula of $C_{11}H_{17}N_3$. It is a colorless prism that in aqueous solution is a mono-acidic base with a pK_a of 8.5. It is only sparingly soluble in water except in a slightly acidic condition, yet at low pH it is not indefinitely stable. In alkaline conditions tetrodotoxin is readily degraded into several quinazoline compounds. The normally high pK_a of the guanidine group of tetrodotoxin is masked by the acidic OH group at C_{10} which has a pK_a of about 8.5. The end NH_2 group enters into formation of a

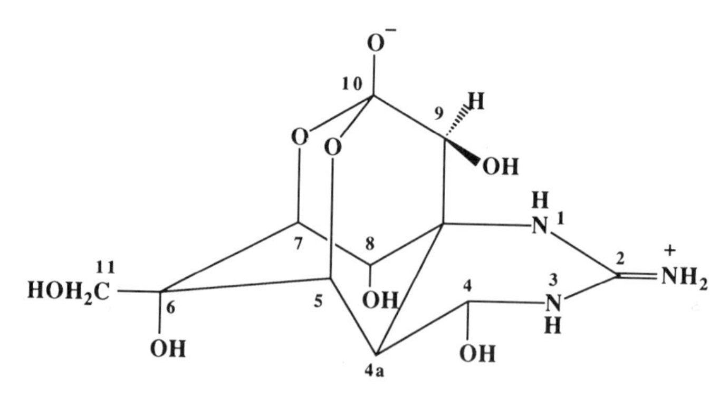

Figure 4.8 Structure of tetrodotoxin.

Zwitterion with one of the OH groups. The toxicities of tetrodotoxin derivatives depend upon the substituent on C_4. The relative lethalities of the derivatives are shown in Table 4.5.

The oxygen link between C_5 and C_{10} in tetrodotoxin seems to be essential if the derivative is to be toxic. This is evident because tetrodonic acid, which does not have this oxygen link, is nontoxic.

F. Ciguatoxin

Toxicologists recognize several forms of ichthyotoxism or fish poisoning (from the Greek root *ichthys*, meaning fish). The word *ciguatera* came from the name cigua which is the name of one of the rollshell species of shellfish, *Cittarium pica*, living in the Caribbean Sea. Ciguatera refers to a widespread and insidious syndrome of ichthyosarcotoxism, that is, toxicity associated with the normally edible skin, viscera, or muscle of fish. More than 400 species of fish have been implicated in ciguatera, including several major food fishes such as barracuda, sea bass, and snapper.

1. *Mode of Toxic Action*

Ciguatera poisoning in humans affects both the gastrointestinal tract and the nervous system. The symptoms of ciguatera are very complex: some victims begin to feel tingling on the lips, tongue, and throat followed by numbness in these areas. In other cases, the initial symptoms consist of nausea, vomiting, a metallic taste, dryness of the mouth, abdominal cramps, diarrhea, headache, prostration, chills, fever, general muscular pain, and so on. Weakness may become progressively worse until the

TABLE 4.5
Relative Lethalities of Tetrodotoxin and Its Derivatives

Compound	Group on C_4[a]	Relative lethality
Tetrodotoxin	$—OH$	1.000
Anhydrotetrodotoxin	$—O—$	0.001
Tetrodaminotoxin	$—NH_2—$	0.010
Methoxytetrodotoxin	$—OCH_3$	0.024
Ethoxytetrodotoxin	$—OC_2H_5$	0.012
Deoxytetrodotoxin	$—H_2$	0.079
Tetrodonic acid	—	0.000

[a] Refer to Figure 4.8.

intoxicated person is unable to walk. Symptoms may persist for a period of a few hours to several weeks and sometimes longer. Death occasionally results, usually a few days after the onset of symptoms. Most reported incidents of fatal human ciguatera poisoning involve barracuda, but the frequency of human poisoning is not known. Ciguatera is believed to be widely underreported throughout the tropical regions of the world and its symptoms are often confused with organophosphate poisoning.

2. *Toxic Principles*

The toxic agent of ciguatera has not been identified; however, some characteristics have been isolated. The toxicity of affected fish is not altered by heating or freezing. There is also some evidence that the toxin can accumulate in humans so that repeated exposure to low levels can result in poisoning. Given the episodic and widely dispersed incidence of this syndrome, as well as the variation in duration of symptoms, it is probable that several toxins, possibly of different origin, are involved. At least four toxic substances, ranging widely in both molecular weight and chemical properties, have been isolated from ciguatoxic fish, but the structures of these compounds have not yet been elucidated.

Various microorganisms have been implicated as the source of ciguatera toxins. These include blue-green algae, Gymnodinium species of dinoflagellates, and marine bacteria. Most ciguatoxic fish are either bottom dwellers or predatory species feeding on bottom dwellers. As with PSP, the toxins do not appear to have any ill effects on the fish. Larger fish of a given species are often proportionately more toxic than smaller fish, suggesting that the toxin can accumulate in fish.

Several methods have been developed to identify ciguatoxic fish. These include bioassays utilizing mice and brine shrimp, radioimmunoassay, and more recently, an enzyme-linked immunoassay. Immunoassay procedures offer both more sensitivity and selectivity than bioassays. However, until all of the toxins responsible for ciguatera have been established, a single immunoassay cannot be considered satisfactory for the protection of public health. Ciguatera has been a serious problem for many years for people living in the islands of the South Pacific and it is also a major barrier to the search for new protein sources from marine resources.

Suggestions for Further Reading

1. World Health Organization. (1984). "Aquatic (Marine and Freshwater) Biotoxins." WHO Publications Centre USA, Albany, New York.

2. Conning, D. M., and Lansdown, A. B. G. (1983). "Toxic Hazards in Food." Raven Press, New York.
3. Graham, H. (ed.) (1980). "The Safety of Foods," 2nd Ed. AVI Publishing Company, Westport, Connecticut.
4. Kato, K., Ohgaki, H., Hasegawas, H., Sato, S., Takayama, S., and Sugimura, T. (1988). Carcinogenicity in rats of a mutagenic compound, 2-amino-3,8-dimethylimidazone[4,5]-quinoaxaline. *Carcinogenesis* **9,** 71.
5. Miller, K. (ed.) (1987). "Toxicological Aspects of Food." Elsevier Applied Science, New York.
6. Ragalis, E. P. (ed.) (1984). "Seafood Toxins." Proceeding of a Symposium of the Division of Agricultural and Food Chemistry at the 186th meeting of the American Chemical Society, American Chemical Society, Washington, D.C.
7. Rechcigl, M., Jr. (ed.) (1983). "CRC Handbook of Naturally Occurring Food Toxicants." CRC Press, Boca Raton, Florida.
8. Searle, C. (ed.) (1976). "Chemical Carcinogens." ACS Monograph 173. American Chemical Society, Washington, D.C.
9. Stauric, B. (ed.) (1974). Mutagenic food flavonoids. *Fed. Proc.* **43,** 2454.
11. Taylor, S. L., and Scanlan, R. A. (ed.) (1989). "Food Toxicology: A Perspective on the Relative Risks." Dekker, New York.
12. Watson, D. H. (ed.) (1987). "Natural Toxicants in Food: Progress and Prospects." VCH Publishers, New York.
13. Weyland, E., and Bevan, D. (1987) Species differences in disposition of benzo[*a*]pyrene. *Drug Metab. Disposition* **15,** 442.

CHAPTER 5

Natural Toxins in Plant Foodstuffs

Since food plants are mixtures of large numbers of chemical compounds and since any substance is toxic in a high enough dose, it is not suprising that natural food plants are toxic under certain conditions. Toxicity from common natural foods has resulted from long-term consumption of a single food item or from short periods of consumption of foods containing unusually high levels of a toxic substance. The process of diet selection has been continuous since prehistory and has minimized consumption of foods of high toxicity.

I. Natural Goitrogens

Human goiter remains a significant problem in certain parts of the world. Only about 4% of human goiter is thought to be due to causes other than iodine deficiency. The cause of endemic goiter may often be interactions of factors such as iodine deficiency and certain food components. In some areas of the world, dietary cruciferous plants could be one of the contributing factors.

Methods of determining the goitrogenic activity of a substance have improved greatly over the years. The earliest method involved visually inspecting and weighing the thyroid glands of experimental animals fed the test substance. More recently, histological examinations of the glands have been used to provide additional information about the nature of the agents or the conditions that cause enlargement. Other criteria used to assess goitrogenic activity are growth rate of the test animal, basal metabolic rates, and assays for iodine content of the thyroid and blood. Current tests consist of measuring the uptake of radioactive iodine by the thyroid gland following feeding of the test material. This procedure has been used with rats, chicks, and humans, and the anti-thyroid response to a substance has been shown to vary with species. Advantages of this test over previous tests are its increased speed and sensitivity. A disadvantage is that the test gives no information on the cumulative anti-thyroid effects of feeding low levels of goitrogen-containing natural products. Examination of this aspect of the problem requires extended administration of the test material, usually in feed of known iodine content, followed by an examination of the thyroid glands.

Goiter can be consistently induced in animals when the seeds of certain Brassica species are included in the feed. However, thyroid enlargement is variable and does not occur when the leafy portion of the vegetable is included in the feed. It is unlikely that consumption of Brassica plants as a normal part of an otherwise adequate diet will induce thyroid enlargement. However, it seems plausible that consumption of unusually large amounts of some of these plants (such as cabbage) might cause thyroid abnormalities. In particular, consumption of Brassica might have contributed to the relatively high incidence of goiter in areas of the world where the dietary iodine intake is low.

The goitrogenic substances in Cruciferae such as goitrin, of which family Brassica is a genus, are formed from glucosinolates (Figure 5.1). These substances may be converted to several products following the action of the enzyme thioglucosidase, which is present in all plants that contain glucosinolates and in certain microorganisms, including gut bacteria. Products of this reaction include nitriles, thiocyanates, and oxazolidines.

The oxazolidine goitrin is a thyroid-suppressing substance as measured by reduced uptake of radioactive iodine and by thyroid enlargement in animals. The racemic mixture of R- and S-goitrin has biological activity equivalent to that of pure goitrin in either optically active form. The activity of goitrin is species-dependent and shows 133% of the activity in man of propylthiouracil, and anti-thyroid drug. Goitrin has relatively weak anti-thyroid activity in rats since long-term feeding of goitrin at 0.23% of the diet causes only mild thyroid enlargement.

Thiocyanate (SCN—) may occur in plants chiefly as a product of glucosinolate and isothiocyanate breakdown. Thyroid enlargement by thiocyanate results from inhibition of iodine uptake by the thyroid gland and is magnified with iodine deficiency.

The mixed nitrile fraction or modified Brassica meals known to con-

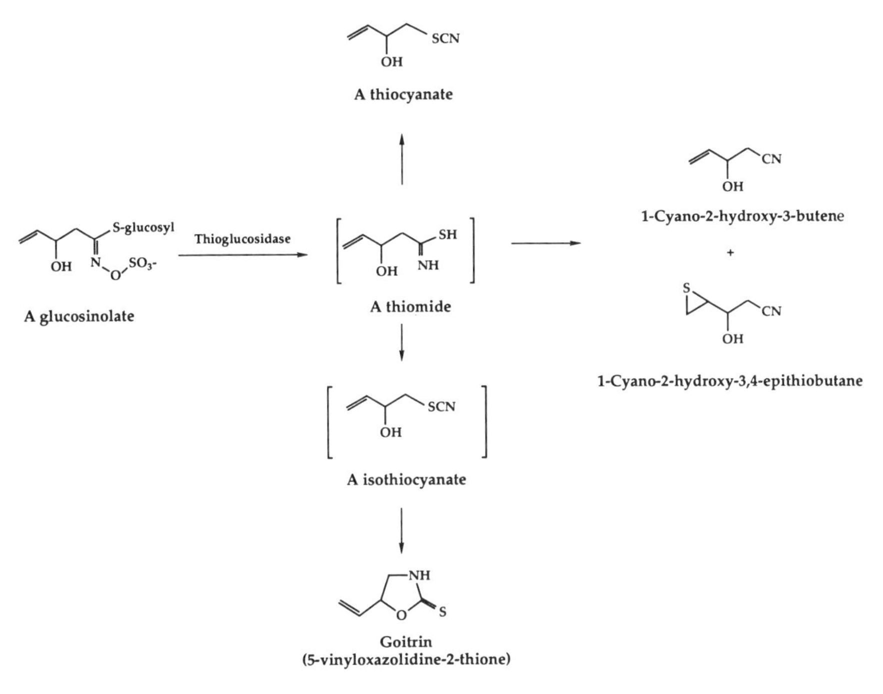

Figure 5.1 Glucosinolate compounds and their formation pathways.

tain a mixture of nitriles are of established toxicity to rats. The toxicities of these nitriles are increased apparently because of the presence of more reactive moieties such as the epithio– or allylic–alcohol components. Such structural components predispose these compounds to nucleophilic attack by key cellular substances, which may result in toxic effects.

Goitrogenic levels of goitrin and thiocyanate are not likely to occur in cow's milk. However, these substances in the feed of cows appear to reduce iodine uptake by the mammary gland, which results in production of milk low in iodine. Thus, milk low in iodine may contribute to goiter development in people heavily dependent on milk as a primary iodine source.

A. Mode of Toxic Action

Secretion of the thyroid hormones thyroxine and triiodothyronine is regulated by the hypothalamus and the pituitary gland in the following manner. The hypothalamus produces thyrotropin-releasing hormone

(TRH) which stimulates the pituitary gland to synthesize and release the thyroid-stimulating hormone (TSH). TSH promotes the uptake of iodine by the thyroid, the synthesis of thyroglobulin, and the release of thyroxine and triiodothyronine. Increased concentrations of the thyroid hormones reduce TSH secretion by a negative feedback mechanism. Alterations in the output of these thyroid hormones result in important changes in oxygen consumption, cardiovascular function, cholesterol metabolism, neuromuscular activity, and cerebral function. Growth and development are also seriously affected when the production of thyroid hormones is deficient. Triiodothyronine is four times as active metabolically as thyroxine. In humans, triiodothyronine is responsible for two-thirds of the biological activity of the thyroid hormones and thyroxine accounts for one-third of the activity.

Several steps are recognized in the synthesis of thyroid hormones. They include

1. concentration of inorganic iodide (iodine trapping);
2. oxidation of iodide to free iodine or hypoiodite;
3. formation of monoiodotyrosine and diiodotyrosine; and
4. coupling of two dioodotyrosines to form thyroxine (tetraiodothyronine).

Enzymes in the liver, kidney, and other organs remove one iodine atom from thyroxine and convert it to triiodothyronine. It is believed that more than half of all circulating triiodothyronine is made by peripheral deiodination of thyroxine and only about one-third is secreted by the thyroid gland.

Substances that depress thyroid function may be placed into one of several categories on the basis of their mode of action. Substances such as goitrin and thiourea inhibit thyroxine synthesis. Substances such as thiocyanates and nitrites inhibit iodide uptake by the thyroid gland through a mechanism that is poorly understood. Substances which inhibit thyroxine synthesis (i.e., goitrin) do not diminish the iodide-concentrating ability of the thyroid gland, but rather block formation of the iodinated amino acids. These substances inhibit thyroxine peroxidase, the iodide oxidizing enzymes. They block the reactions that require free iodine. When substances in this group of inhibitors of thyroxine synthesis are administered to humans or experimental animals, the performed thyroxine continues to be secreted. However, thyroxine secretion diminishes as the stored organic iodine becomes exhausted because of lack of resynthesis. This causes increased secretion of the TSH, which produces a hyperplastic, highly vascularized thyroid gland that has a greatly increased capacity for iodide trapping.

II. Cyanogenic Glycosides

Cyanogenic glycosides are a group of widely occurring natural substances that on hydrolysis yield a ketone or aldehyde, a sugar, and the highly toxic cyanide ion. Toxicity of cyanogenic glycosides is due to the liberation of cyanide (see Table 5.1 for the major food and feed sources of cyanide). Cyanide release from cyanogenic glycosides occurs readily in the laboratory by acid or base hydrolysis. However, hydrogen cyanide release is not appreciable in the stomach in spite of the decidedly acidic nature of its contents. Hydrogen cyanide is released from cyanogenic glycosides in chewed or chopped plants or following ingestion by an enzymatic process involving two enzymes (Figure 5.2). The first step is cleavage of the sugar, catalyzed by β-glucosidase, which yields a cyanohydrin and a sugar. Most cyanohydrins are relatively unstable and spontaneously decompose to the corresponding ketone or aldehyde and hydrogen cyanide. However, this decomposition is accelerated by the action of the enzyme, hydroxynitrile lyase. The cyanogenic glycoside and the enzymes necessary for release of hydrogen cyanide are all present but separated in the plant. When fresh plant material is macerated as in chewing, cell structures are broken down sufficiently to allow the enzymes and the cyanogenic glycoside to come into contact to produce hydrogen cyanide. This is thought to be the principal mechanism of cyanide poisoning from consumption of fresh plant material.

Several methods, including chopping and grinding, have been developed to detoxify cyanogenic food products. In practice, cassava, which is an important source of carbohydrate for people in South America and Africa, is most often chopped and ground in running water, a process which can remove both cyanogenic glycosides and any released hydrogen cyanide. Fermentation and boiling processes are also used in the production of cassava flour. In spite of this well-developed processing procedure,

TABLE 5.1
Food Sources of Cyanogenic Glycosides and Amount of HCN Produced

Plant	Amount of HCN (mg/100 g)	Glucoside
Bitter almonds	250	Amygdalin
Cassava root	53	Linamarin
Sorghum (whole plant)	250	Dhurrin
Lima bean	10–312	Linamarin

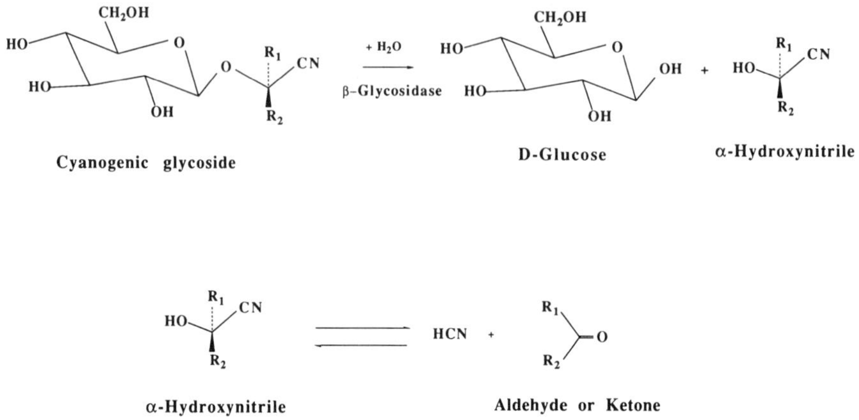

Cyanogenic glycoside $\xrightarrow[\beta\text{-Glycosidase}]{+H_2O}$ D-Glucose + α-Hydroxynitrile

α-Hydroxynitrile ⇌ HCN + Aldehyde or Ketone

Figure 5.2 The release of hydrogen cyanide from cyanogenic glycosides.

the cyanide content of cassava products can remain significant. In general, the more extensively purified cassava flours are the most expensive, which generally forces individuals with limited financial resources to depend on the more heavily contaminated flour as a food.

Purified cyanogenic glycosides or cyanogenic glycosides in food that has been boiled to inactivate enzymes produce somewhat variable toxic effects in animals and people. Purified cyanogenic glycosides, i.e., amygdalin, fed to guinea pigs in very large doses produced no toxic effect. Although cyanogenic glycosides are stable in saliva and gastric juices, consumption of twice-boiled lima beans known to contain cyanogenic glycosides produces symptoms of acute cyanide poisoning, and lima beans boiled for 2.5 hr induces vomiting and increased levels of urinary cyanide. This evidence indicates that people may harbor intestinal organisms that contain the enzymes necessary to free cyanide from ingested cyanogenic glycosides.

A. Cyanide Toxicity

Cyanide is considered a highly toxic substance. Symptoms of acute poisoning include mental confusion, muscular paralysis, and respiratory distress. The minimal lethal oral dose of hydrogen cyanide is estimated to be 0.5–3.5 mg/kg body weight. Cyanide exerts its toxic effects by binding to the ferric ion of cytochrome oxidase in mitochondria. The overall effect is cessation of cellular respiration.

The cyanide ion is normally metabolized as indicated in Figure 5.3. The principal excretion product of cyanide is thiocyanate, the production of which is catalyzed by rhodenase, an enzyme that is widely occurring in most mammalian tissues. Minor metabolic routes of cyanide involve reaction with cysteine to produce a thiazoline and an oxidative pathway leading ultimately to carbon dioxide and formate. An additional minor metabolic pathway for cyanide is complication with hydroxycobalamin. This complication may be the normal metabolic route of small amounts of cyanide in the body.

The usual treatment for acute cyanide poisoning is administration of nitrite or nitrite esters such as amyl nitrite, which converts hemoglobin (Fe^{2+}) to methemoglobin (Fe^{3+}). Increased circulating levels of methemoglobin will draw cyanide away from cytochrome oxidase, thus allowing cellular respiration to proceed. Final detoxification of the cyanide is facilitated by administration of thiosulfate required for formation of thiocyanate.

Although the effects of acute cyanide poisoning are fairly well-defined, the results of chronic cyanide poisoning are less well established. Consumption of cassava in certain parts of Africa and South America is associated with at least two disorders that do not seem to occur in areas where cassava consumption is low or in individuals who consume cassava free of cyanide. A disorder known as tropical ataxic neuropathy (TAN)

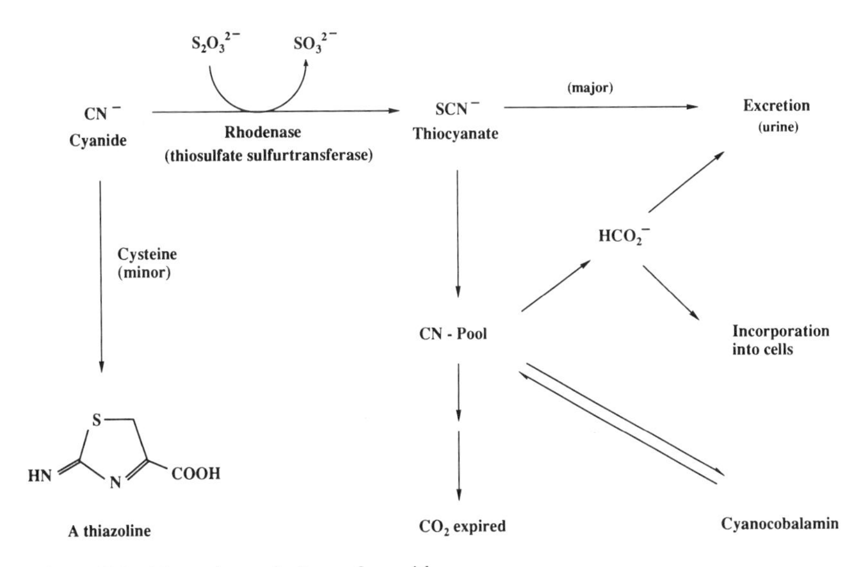

Figure 5.3 Normal metabolism of cyanide.

and characterized by optic atrophy, ataxia, and mental disorder is found in areas of West Africa where cassava is a staple of the diet. Individuals with this disorder have very low concentrations of sulfur amino acids in the blood and elevated levels of plasma thiocyanate. Symptoms of the disease subside when patients are placed on cyanide–free diets and recur when traditional eating habits are resumed. Goiter is also prevalent in these areas. This is not surprising in view of the elevated blood levels of thiocyanate, an established goitrogen.

A related syndrome that is associated with prolonged consumption of cyanide is known as tropical amblyopia. This disease, characterized by atrophy of the optic nerve, resulting in blindness, is prevalent in populations consuming cassava as a staple in the diet. Long-term administration of sublethal doses of cyanide to animals results in destruction of optic nerve tissue. Similar effects have been seen in people exposed to low concentrations of cyanide for long periods of time.

The toxic effects of chronic cyanide consumption are modified by other dietary components, and cyanide-induced goiter is not observed if the diet has adequate levels of iodine. Cyanide-induced neurological destruction is generally seen only in partially malnourished populations. The ultimate source of sulfur required for conversion of cyanide to thiocyanate is sulfur-containing amino acids. Diets deficient in these substances result in a decreased ability to detoxify cyanide and increased circulating levels of cyanide. Chronic consumption of cyanide in marginally protein-deficient diets can magnify the sulfur deficiency of these diets. Thus, consumption of foods containing cyanogenic glycosides may not only result in toxic effect directly attributable to cyanide, but may indirectly promote effects characteristic of protein malnutrition.

III. Favism

Favism is a syndrome of acute hemolytic anemia induced by consumption of raw or cooked Vicia fava beans, commonly known as broad beans or fava beans. Favism is generally restricted to populations near the Mediterranean Sea or in China. The disease occurs to a greater extent in males than in females and is more severe in infants and young children than in adults. While adult deaths from favism rarely occur, fatalities have been reported in infants and children. The clinical symptoms of favism may include pallor, fatigue, shortness of breath, nausea, abdominal pain, fever, and chills. Renal failure occurs in the more severe cases. The onset of symptoms generally occurs within 24 hr following ingestion of the bean and persists for up to 2 days. Recovery in most individuals is spontaneous and abrupt.

Studies of the etiology of favism have been hampered by the unavailability of a suitable animal model for the disease. However, the results of several epidemiologic studies indicate that susceptible individuals have decreased levels of both glucose-6-phosphate-dehydrogenase (G6PD) and reduced glutathione (GSH) in red blood cells. G6PD catalyzes a reaction in glucose metabolism that produces NADPH. Adequate levels of GSH in turn are maintained by the glutathione reductase-mediated reaction of oxidized glutathione (GSSG) with NADPH. Thus, reduced levels of G6PD result in a diminished capacity of cells to maintain normal levels of GSH. Adequate levels of GSH, an antioxidant, are required to maintain stability of the cell membrane.

In experiments with suspensions of human red blood cells, it was found that GSH levels of cells from individuals susceptible to favism are affected by components of the fava bean included in the suspension mixture. GSH levels of cells from normal individuals do not show this sensitivity. The active substances in fava bean are pyrimidine derivatives, divicine, and isouramil, which are the corresponding aglycones of vicine and convicine (Figure 5.4). These aglycones are readily oxidized in air and rapidly promote the nonenzymatic conversion of GSH to GSSG in solution. Thus, it is suggested that these pyrimidine derivatives formed from the corresponding glycosides by enzymatic action in the plant or in the gut may be causative agents of favism. Confirmation of this hypothesis must await development of a suitable animal model for the disease or appropriate tests in humans.

IV. Lathyrism

Lathyrism is an ancient disease caused by consumption of certain peas of the genus *Lathyrus,* known as vetch peas, chick-peas, or garbanzos. The disease is primarily restricted to areas of India where epidemics of the disease still occur. Although *L. sativus* is well known to be toxic and its cultivation and sale in most parts of India are banned, its hardiness under adverse growing conditions and its resistance to drought make it a sought-after crop. Lathyrism has two manifestations, osteolathyrism and neurolathyrism.

Osteolathyrism is a disease seen in animals consuming various lathyrus species. The disease is characterized by bone deformations and weakness in aeortic and connective tissue. Although many substances

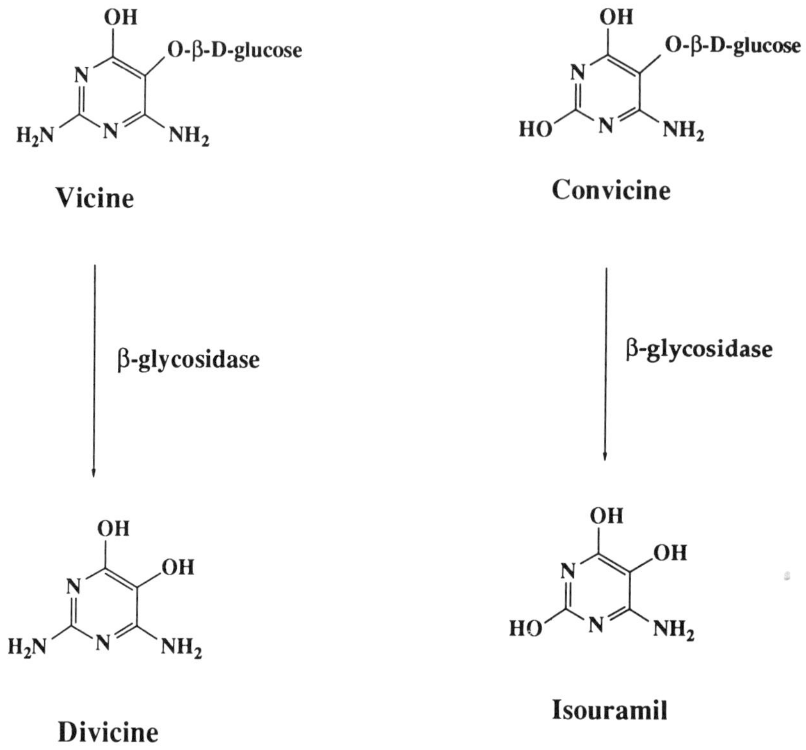

Vicine   Convicine

β-glycosidase   β-glycosidase

Divicine   Isouramil

Figure 5.4 Structures of the active substances in fava bean.

have been tested and found to have osteolathyrogenic activity, the lathyrogenic activity of lathyrus species seems to be restricted to a single substance, *β*-L-glutamylaminopropionitrile (BAPN, Figure 5.5). When BAPN was included in the diet of rats at the level of 0.1–0.2%, skeletal deformity and aeortic rupture developed.

The mode of action of BAPN in osteolathyrism has been studied in some detail. The principal effect of BAPN is to inhibit the cross-linking of collagen, the primary structural protein of connective tissue and bone. Collagen cross-linking requires an initial oxidative deamination of peptide bound lysine, catalyzed by the enzyme lysyl oxidase. The oxidized lysine residues combine with amino acids on adjacent peptide chains, forming the insoluble cross-linked collagen. BAPN irreversibly inhibits lysyl oxidase, thus preventing the formation of the collagen network.

Neurolathyrism is the form of the lathyrus-induced disease that affects humans. The disease, caused by long-term consumption (longer

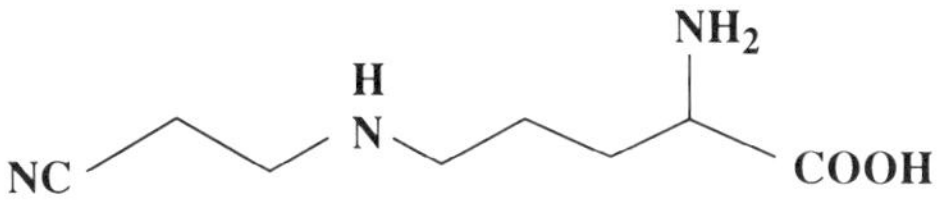

NH_2
H
N
NC COOH

Figure 5.5 Structure of BAPN.

than 3 months) of *L. sativus*, is characterized by increasing paralysis of the legs, followed by general weakness and muscular rigidity. The onset of the symptoms is often sudden and may be initiated with a sudden contraction of the calf muscles of the leg. Most cases of the disease involve young men.

Studies of the etiology of neurolathyrism have been hampered in the past by the inability to reproduce this disease in laboratory animals. In initial studies, crude extracts, purified fractions from *L. sativus*, were tested for activity by injection into day-old chicks. Toxic reactions include convulsions and other reactions indicative of neurological damage. In these early studies, β-*N*-oxalyl-L-α,β-diaminopropionic acid (OPAP, Figure 5.6), which is absent in other species of Lathyrus, was isolated from *L. sativus*. ODAP produced neurological responses in young rats, young guinea pigs, and young dogs. However, neurological symptoms in adult rats could be seen only on injection of ODAP into the brain. Neurologic symptoms have been induced in adult squirrel monkeys by intraperitoneal injection, and selective concentration of ODAP in the cerebellum of these monkeys was noted. Thus, although a role of ODAP as the causative agent in human neurolathyrism has not been proven, the data accumulated in studies with animals support this hypothesis.

The mechanism by which ODAP exerts its toxic effect on the nervous system has not been established. However, there is increasing evidence that ODAP may interfere with the normal function of glutamic acid at the nerve synapse. ODAP competitively inhibits the uptake of glutamic acid into the cells of various microorganisms. ODAP also inhibits the uptake of glutamic acid by synaptic components of rat and monkey nervous systems. Release of glutamic acid from these synaptic components is enhanced, however, following treatment with ODAP. Thus, the

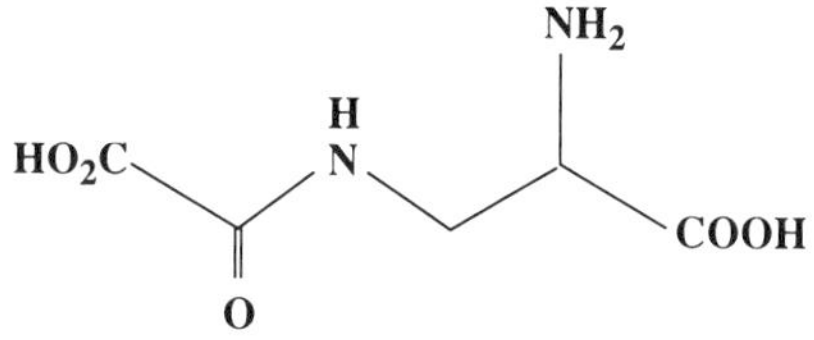

NH_2
H
HO_2C N
COOH
O

Figure 5.6 Structure of ODAP.

overall effect of ODAP appears to be a net increase of glutamic acid concentration at the synapse. The significance of this increase in terms of the toxic lesions of neurolathyrism remains to be determined.

V. Lectins (Hemagglutinins)

Lectins are a rather remarkable group of proteins and glycoproteins that possess the ability to bind certain carbohydrates. When these carbohydrates are components of cell walls, lectins will cause the agglutination of the cells which contain them. The ability of lectins to agglutinate red blood cells is used as a basis for assays of blood types. When lectins bind to carbohydrate components of intestinal epithelial cells, the result may be a decreased absorption of nutrients from the digestive tract.

Lectins are widely distributed in nature. Extracts from over 800 plant species and from numerous animal species show agglutinating activity. Of particular interest here are the lectins that occur in various legumes used as feed or food sources. Lectin activity has been shown to occur in a wide variety of legumes used for food such as black beans, soybeans, lima beans, kidney beans, peas, and lentils.

Although lectins are a group of substances which have been recognized because of their ability to agglutinate or clump red blood cells, some of these substances are also highly toxic to animals. For example, lectins isolated from black beans produce growth retardation when fed to rats at 0.5% of the diet, and lectin from kidney beans produces death in rats fed on lectin at 0.5% of the diet for 2 weeks. Soybean lectin, a less toxic lectin, fed at 1% of the diet to rats produces only growth retardation. The LD_{50} of soybean lectin is estimated as 50 mg/kg. Ricin, a lectin from the castor bean, is one of the most toxic natural substances with an LD_{50} by injection of 0.05 mg/kg. Because of their high toxicity, castor beans (not a legume) must be thoroughly heated to deactivate their ricin before they can be used as animal feed.

The exact role of lectins in the anti-nutritional or toxic effects of various beans and legumes is the subject of some controversy and appears to depend on the specific legume in question. Uncooked beans as a major component of the diet generally do not support the growth of animals. Thoroughly heated beans, of course, do support growth. When the lectin fractions of black beans and kidney beans are fed to animals along with the heated bean material, toxic symptoms are manifested. In the case of soybeans, about half of the growth depression caused by raw soy meal can be attributed to the lectin. In addition, little improvement in nutritional quality is observed for soybean meal from which the lectin component has been removed. Thus, in addition to lectins, other substances such as inhibitors of digestive enzymes appear to contribute to the growth-depressing effects of raw beans.

The mechanism by which lectins produce an ultimate toxic effect is also open to controversy. It is well established that lectins from various sources present on the intestinal epithelium adsorb nutrients and thus reduce the absorption of those nutrients by the intestine. The resulting inefficient use of nutrients may in itself account for the poor growth promoted by diets rich in uncooked legumes. This effect may also magnify the protein losses induced by pancreatic hypersecretion caused by trypsin inhibitors also present in the legumes (see following). However, the microflora of the gut also appear to play a role in legume- and lectin-induced toxicity. Germ-free birds (i.e., birds free of intestinal bacteria) used as test species show less growth depression when fed raw legumes or isolated lectins than do conventional birds. For example, diets containing raw jack beans meal produce high mortality in Japanese quail. However, germ-free birds exhibit no toxic effects under exactly the same experimental conditions; these observations have led some investigators to suggest that the lectins may impair the body's defense system against bacterial infection, resulting in an increased tendency for an invasion by gut and other bacterial flora.

VI. Pyrrolizidine Alkaloids

The pyrrolizidine alkaloids (Figure 5.7) are a group of substances of related structure produced by a variety of plants, including many range plants (*Senecio, Crotalaria, Heliotropium*) that are consumed by livestock. Over 100 pyrrolizidine alkaloids have been isolated from various plants, and the levels range from traces up to 5% of the dry weight of the plant. Some of the compounds are potent carcinogens. Administration of one of the plants, *Senecio longilobus*, at 0.5% of the diet every other week

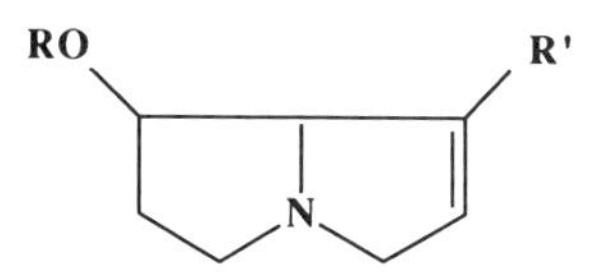

Figure 5.7 Structure of pyrrolizidine alkaloids.

induced tumors in 17 of 47 rats that survived the test. The doses of pure compounds required to induce carcinogenesis are moderately high, however. In one experiment, the pyrrolizidine alkaloid, monocrotaline, was given intragastrically to rats once a week at a dose of 25 mg/kg for 4 weeks, then at 7 mg/kg body weight for 38 weeks. This regimen induced cancers in approximately 25% of the animals treated. In another experiment, weekly intraperitoneal injections of lasiocarpine at a dose of 7.8 mg/kg body weight for 1 year produced no tumors. However, following this year of treatment, a high percentage of the survivors developed malignant tumors of the skin, bones, liver, and other organs.

It is not certain whether these substances are passed along to humans in products such as milk and meat. Some of the pyrrolizidine-containing plants are used in herbal remedies and for tea preparations. In addition, one species of comfrey, known to contain pyrrolizidine alkaloids, is used as a green vegetable in Japan. However, the importance of pyrrolizidine alkaloids in human carcinogenesis is as yet unclear.

The carcinogenic and mutagenic activity of pyrrolizidine alkaloids is dependent on metabolism to an ultimate, reactive form. The presence of the 1,2-double bond in the pyrrolizidine nucleus appears to be required for carcinogenic activity. The exact role of this double bond has not been determined with certainty, although epoxidation at this site is a likely possibility. The resulting epoxide is then subject to nucleophilic attack. However, the 1,2-double bond also facilitates dehydrogenation to the corresponding pyrrole, which may also be subject to nucleophilic attack.

VII. Enzyme Inhibitors

Detection of biological activity is, of course, dependent on the development of an appropriate bioassay. For reasons of sensitivity, convenience, and cost, most bioassays incorporate some *in vitro* techniques. It is important to remember, however, that this *in vitro* activity may not be relevant to biological effects *in vivo*. While it is true that the hemagglutinating activity of the lectins discussed in a previous section has been used in blood type determinations, this activity is of little importance to the toxicity of some of these substances *in vivo*. Another readily determined property of foods or their components is their ability to inhibit certain enzyme-mediated reactions. Bioassays for this type of activity generally require incubation of a specific enzyme and its substrate along with the substance to be tested. The importance of enzyme activity to the potential toxicity of a food or food component is not always clear. In this section protease inhibitors and cholinesterase inhibitors will be discussed.

A. Protease Inhibitors

Inhibitors of enzymes involved in the hydrolysis of protein (protease inhibitors) are widespread throughout the plant kingdom. Legumes are a major source of these substances, although they also occur in other foods. Inhibitors of trypsin, a gastric protease, have been isolated from most varieties of legumes and grains as well as from other foods such as potatoes, eggplant, and onions.

Indications that trypsin inhibitors play a role in the anti-nutritional properties of certain legumes come from animal experiments. The growth of several species of laboratory animals is inhibited by anti-tryptic components from beans. Addition of purified trypsin inhibitors to diets containing predigested protein or amino acids causes an obvious growth retardation in rodents. However, the protease-inhibitory effect of these substances does not appear to be the cause of the decreased growth rate. In addition to the growth-retardant effect of the trypsin inhibitors, pancreatic hypertrophy is observed in some animal species. The attendant hypersecretion of pancreatic enzymes combined with the marginal levels of certain essential amino acids in soy protein are a possible cause of the anti-nutritional effects of raw beans. Selective removal of the trypsin inhibitor results in a 40% decrease in the pancreatic hypertrophic effect of the original raw beans. In addition, supplementation of raw soy meal with certain amino acids eliminates the growth-depressing effect of raw meal while not affecting the pancreatic hypertrophic effect. Thus, it appears that the pancreatic hypersecretion of proteins rich in amino acids that are marginal in the diet results in amino acid deficiency and attendant growth depression.

B. Cholinesterase Inhibitors

Cholinesterase is an enzyme that mediates hydrolysis of acetylcholine to acetate and choline. Acetylcholine, present in vesicles in the axonal terminus, is the substance responsible for transmisison of the nerve impulse across the synapse. Stimulation of the vesticles causes the release of acetylcholine, which diffuses across the synapse and initiates the impulse in the adjacent neuron. Once the nerve impulse is transmitted, the acetylcholine must be hydrolyzed so that the neuron can be repolarized in preparation for the next impulse.

Some plants contain compounds that inhibit cholinesterase activity, of which undoubtedly the most notorious plant is the West African calibar bean. This bean is the source of physostigmine (Figure 5.8), a potent

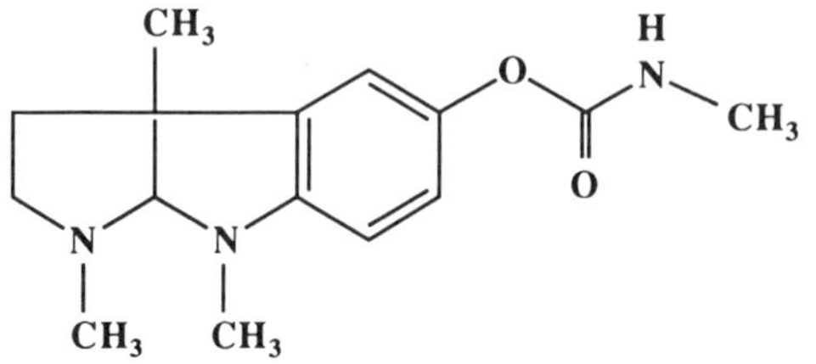

Figure 5.8 Structure of physostigmine.

cholinesterase inhibitor and a model for the carbamate class of insecticides. Preparations of this highly toxic and inedible bean have been used as an ordeal poison in witchcraft trials in Africa.

The anticholinesterase substance found in food products that has perhaps been studied the most is solanine (Figure 5.9), a glycosidal alkaloid (glycoalkaloid) composed of a carbohydrate residue and the aglycone, solanidine. Solanine is found primarily in members of the genus *Solanum,* which includes eggplant, potato, and tomato.

The total glycoalkaloid content of potato tubers varies with the variety and appears to be within the range of 20 to 100 mg/kg of fresh tissue. However, a variety (Lenape) developed for potato chips had a total glycoalkaloid content of about 300 mg/kg fresh tuber. The use of Lenape as a food product was discontinued. Glycoalkaloid levels of over 200 mg/kg fresh weight are now considered excessive and potentially dangerous. The FDA prohibits the sale of food products containing these levels.

Although solanine is found throughout the potato tuber, the greatest concentrations occur in the sprouts, peelings, and sun-greened areas. In the sprouts, solanine represents about 40% of the total glycoalkaloids, with another similar compound, chaconine, comprising 60%. Chaconine differs from solanine only in the composition of the carbohydrate moiety.

Greening of the potatoes, whether by natural or artificial light, can considerably increase the levels of glycoalkaloids. For example, 5 days of exposure to white fluorescent light will increase the total glycoalkaloid content in the peel of a Russet Burbank variety from approximately 250 to 700 mg/kg. The green appearance of these potatoes is due to increased chlorophyll content which in itself is not hazardous.

Consumption of potatoes by people or animals occasionally has been reported to cause illness or death. Poisoning has resulted from ingestion of potato sprouts, sprouted potatoes, and greened potatoes. In one instance of human poisoning involving six people, the symptoms were described as increasing gastric pain followed by nausea and vomiting.

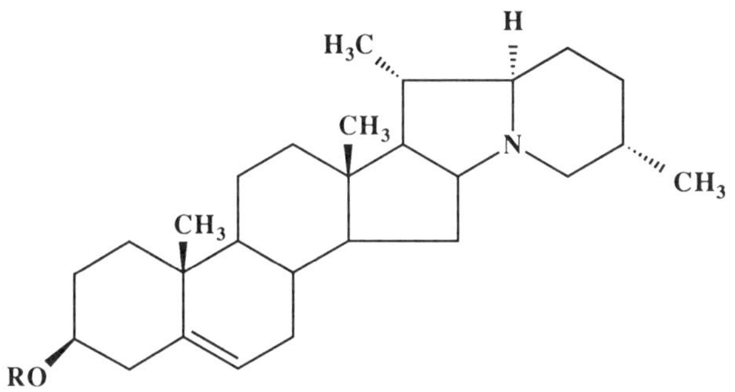

Solanidine: R = H
Solanine: R = Galactosyl - glucosyl - rhamnosyl
Chaconine: R = Glycosyl - rhamnosyl - rhamnosyl

Figure 5.9 Structures of solanidine and related compounds.

Respiration was difficult and accelerated with market weakness and prostration. In this instance, two people died approximately 1 week after consumption of the greened potatoes. Experimental solanine poisoning induced in human volunteers yields symptoms similar to those reported in the case of green potato poisoning. Doses of approximately 3 mg/kg caused drowsiness, itchiness in the neck region, increased sensitivity (hyperesthesia), and labored breathing. Higher doses caused vomiting and diarrhea. Gastrointestinal symptoms (abdominal pain, nausea, vomiting, and diarrhea) are also observed in human intoxication by organophosphate pesticides, which are potent cholinesterase inhibitors.

Although the symptoms of green-potato poisoning and those of acute solanine toxicity are quite similar and therefore implicate solanine as a causative factor, the level of solanine present in the toxic potatoes apparently is not high enough to produce the toxic symptoms by itself. Total alkaloid content of approximately 420 mg/kg of fresh potato has been determined in two cases of human poisoning from potatoes. With the assumption that total alkaloid is composed of 50% solanine, an individual would be required to consume as much as 1 kg of whole potato in order to approach the 200 mg of solanine determined to induce the initial signs of solanine toxicity. In addition, results of experiments with animals have shown that solanine is a substance of low oral toxicity. Thus, oral LD_{50}'s in sheep, rats, and mice are on the order of 500, 600, and over 1000 mg/kg, respectively. It appears, therefore, that solanine is but one of the causative agents of green-potato poisoning and probably acts in combination with other substances such as chaconine or other possibly minor components of potato. The toxicology of chaconine and other potato components requires further investigation.

VIII. Vasoactive Amines

A wide variety of foods from plant and animal sources contain biologically active amines. Substances such as putrescine and cadaverine (Figure 5.10) may occur in meat and fish products as a result of bacterial action on certain amino acids. Other substances, such as dopamine and tyramine, may occur as natural components of certain food plants such as banana and avocado.

Substances that affect the vascular system are known as vasoactive amines. Vasoactive amines that constrict blood vessels and thereby increase blood pressure are known as pressor amines. The pressor amines, norepinephrine and dopamine (the catecholamines) (Figure 5.10), are important neurotransmitters released from adrenergic nerve cells. One of the many striking biological effects of intravenous administration of

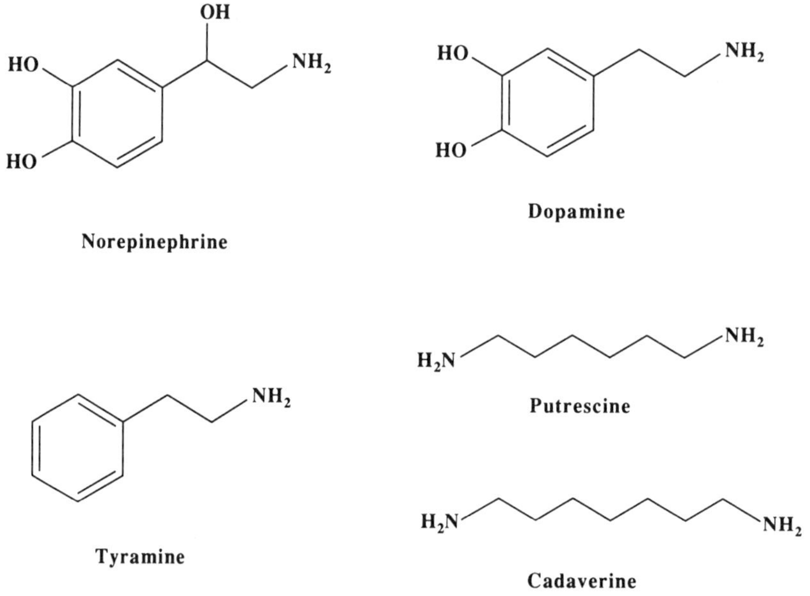

Norepinephrine

Dopamine

Tyramine

Putrescine

Cadaverine

Figure 5.10 Structures of vasoactive amines.

catecholamines in animals is a sharp rise in blood pressure due primarily to direct vasoconstrictive action of these substances. Tyramine, which is not normally a product of mammalian metabolism, can increase blood pressure by an indirect mechanism. Administered tyramine is taken up by the reabsorption process that normally controls intraneuronal levels of catecholamines. This reabsorption of tyramine displaces catecholamines from storage granules, thereby freeing catecholamines with an attendant rise in blood pressure.

Circulating levels of exogenous pressor amines and other vasoactive amines are carefully controlled by the action of monoamine oxidase (MAO), an enzyme of wide distribution in the body. Because of rapid metabolic conversion of amines by MAO and other enzymes, administration of pressor amines to normal mammals generally has little effect on blood pressure. However, marked pressor effects are observed when MAO is inhibited. Certain MAO inhibitors have been used in the clinical treatment of psychiatric depression. Examples of such drugs include isocarboxazid, nialamide, phenylzine sulfate, and tranylcypromine. One of the serious disadvantages of the clinical use of MAO inhibitors is the increased likelihood of adverse reactions to ingested foods that may release monoamines in the body. The ingestion of aged cheese, beer, or certain wines has caused severe hypertensive reactions in patients who were being treated with MAO inhibitors. A listing of amines in certain foods is indicated in Table 5.2. Observed symptoms included hypertensive crisis, migraine headaches, and in some cases, intracranial bleeding leading to death. The cause of these reactions was traced to the presence of tryamine in foods and beverages.

TABLE 5.2
Amine Content of Food Products (in μg/g)

Food product	Serotonin	Tyramine	Dopamine	Norepinephrine
Banana pulp	28	7	8	2
Tomato	12	4	0	0
Avocado	10	23	4–5	0
Potato	0	2	0	0.1–0.2
Spinach	0	1	0	0
Orange	0	10	0	< 0.1
Cheddar cheese	—	120–1500	—	—
Camembert cheese	—	20–2000	—	—
Stilton blue cheese	—	466–2170	—	—
Processed cheese	—	26–50	—	—

IX. Mutagens in Natural Plants

A. Flavonoids

The flavonoids are a group of widely occurring plant substances used to flavor and color foods. One of these substances, quercetin, is the most common flavonoid compound in vascular plants (Figure 5.11). It occurs in conjugated or free form in many plant products such as fruits, vegetables, and teas. Quercetin and its close relative, kaempferol, tested mutagenic in the Ames assay. Quercetin is mutagenic without metabolic activation, but its activity is increased with the incorporation of the liver homogenate into the test system.

Other flavonoids, such as rutin, in which the 3-hydroxyl group of quercetin is conjugated with a carbohydrate, are not mutagenic unless an enzymatic preparation is included in the mixture that hydrolyzes the glycoside linkage. Such an enzymatic mixture is present in the intestines of humans and animals. Long-term feeding studies with quercetin have failed to show that the substance is a carcinogen. On the contrary, quercetin has anticancer properties.

B. Maltoles

Maltol, ethyl maltol (Figure 5.12), and diacetyl are weak mutagens. However, relatively large amounts of the substances are present in the diet. The usual levels of maltol added to baked goods, ice creams, and candy are approximately 110 ppm. Levels on the order of 80 ppm are added to certain beverages. Ethyl maltol, a more potent flavor enhancer than maltol, is generally used in concentrations of about 20 ppm in these foods.

In the United States, the average daily intake of maltol and ethyl

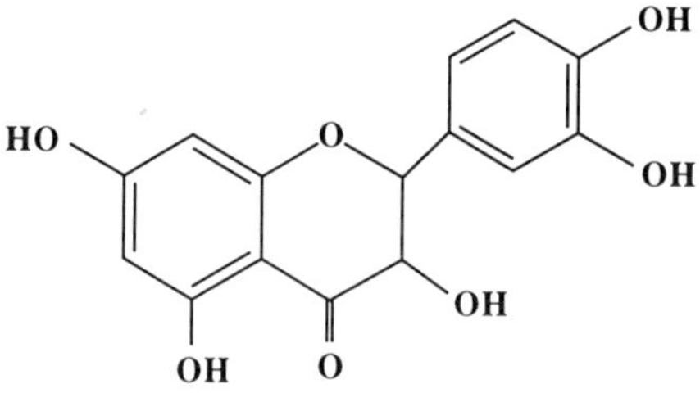

Figure 5.11 Structure of quercetin.

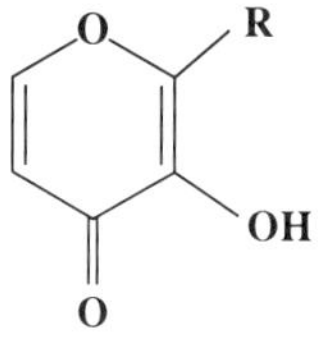

Maltol: R = CH_3

Ethyl maltol: R = C_2H_5

Figure 5.12 Structures of maltole and ethyl maltole.

maltol from all food categories for individuals 2–65 years old is estimated to be 29 and 5 mg, respectively. In certain individuals, the actual levels of consumption may be several times these averages. However, there is no evidence of ill effects in humans from normal dietary consumption of these substances. Results of experiments with dogs indicate that maltol and ethyl maltol are rapidly and efficiently absorbed following oral administration and converted to the glucuronide conjugate. Similar processes probably occur in humans.

Maltol, ethyl maltol, and diacetyl are representatives of the 1,2-dicarbonyl class of chemicals. The total daily human doses of mutagenic 1,2-dicarbonyl compounds are likely to be much greater than estimates based on known levels of maltol, ethyl maltol, and diacetyl. Other 1,2-dicarbonyl compounds such as intermediates in enzymatic and nonenzymatic browning reactions in foods are weakly mutagenic in the Ames test. No conclusive evidence showing the carcinogenic activities of these substances has been presented.

C. Caffeine

Caffeine is a methyladed xanthine derivative (Figure 5.13) that occurs naturally in coffee, tea, cola, and cocoa products. The levels of caffeine in coffee range from 75 to 155 mg per 5-oz cup, with an average of about 115 mg. Traditional teas contain around 40 mg caffeine/cup, and milk chocolate and baking chocolate contain around 6 and 35 mg/oz, respectively. Caffeine is rapidly absorbed from the gastrointestinal tract and distributed throughout the body. It is metabolized and cleared from the blood stream within a few hours in most people. However, clearance rates during pregnancy and in infants are considerably reduced.

Caffeine causes a host of biological effects. At low doses of around 200 mg for an adult, caffeine produces (among other effects) central

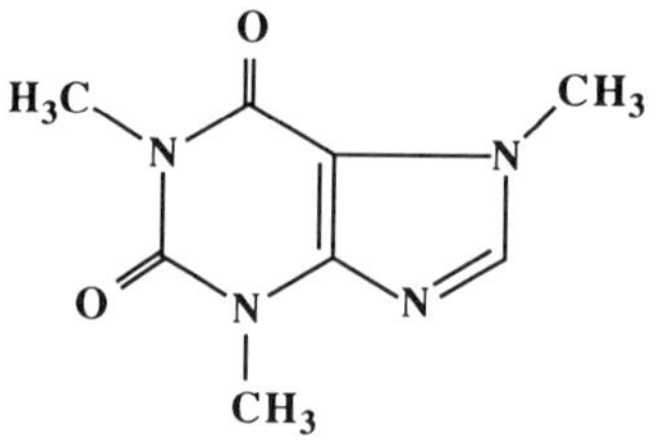

$$\text{Caffeine: 1,3,7-trimethylxanthine structure}$$

Figure 5.13 Structure of caffeine.

nervous system stimulation, diuresis, relaxation of smooth muscles, cardiac muscle stimulation, and increased gastric secretion. The centuries-old belief that caffeine improves physical performance in fatigued individuals has been substantiated scientifically, but performance of rested individuals is not affected by caffeine. Excessive consumption of caffeine can result in nervousness, irritability, and cardiac arrhythmias. The LD_{50} for caffeine is estimated to be 200 mg/kg body weight, which puts caffeine in the moderately toxic range. Under laboratory conditions, caffeine causes many other effects, including teratogenesis, mutagenesis, carcinogenesis, and anticarcinogenesis. Although none of these effects has been substantiated in humans, a panel of the United States National Academy of Sciences has recommended moderation in caffeine consumption for pregnant women.

D. Constituents of Spices

Spices are a prized group of minor components in human diets. The spice trade is one of the oldest trades known and the overland trade routes across the Old World predate recorded history. Spices include a variety of plant products, many with pungent flavors, that are used to enhance the natural flavors and aromas of foods and beverages. Spices often contain substances with potent biological activities. Examples of a few of these substances are discussed in the following section.

1. Onion and Garlic

Human consumption of onion (50–60 g), along with a high-fat diet, prevented both the increased tendency of blood to clot and the rise in serum cholesterol normally seen following the consumption of high-fat diets. Onion and garlic juice and the ether-extractable essential oils of these products have similar effects. Long-term feeding (4 months) of the essential oils of onion and garlic to rabbits decreased cholesterol-induced atherosclerotic lesions of the aorta by about one-half. The striking properties of onion and garlic esssential oils have led some investigators to suggest the use of these products in the treatment of individuals who are predisposed to atherosclerosis and thrombosis. Components of these essential oils also show promise as anticancer agents.

2. *Celery Oil*

Two uses of celery seed oil in folk medicine are as a sedative and as a nerve tonic. Much of the aroma of celery seed oil can be ascribed to the presence of certain phthalides (Figure 5.14), one of which is called sedanolide. Although the name of this compound implies sedative activity, no such studies were actually carried out until fairly recently. Although sedanolide does not appear to be a generally occurring component of celery essential oil, other phthalides (3-*n*-butylphthalide and sedanenolide) are primarily responsible for the odor of this spice. Both of these substances are weak sedatives in mice. Because of the weakness of this activity, however, it appears that consumption of unusually large amounts of celery oil would be required to produce a sedative effect in people.

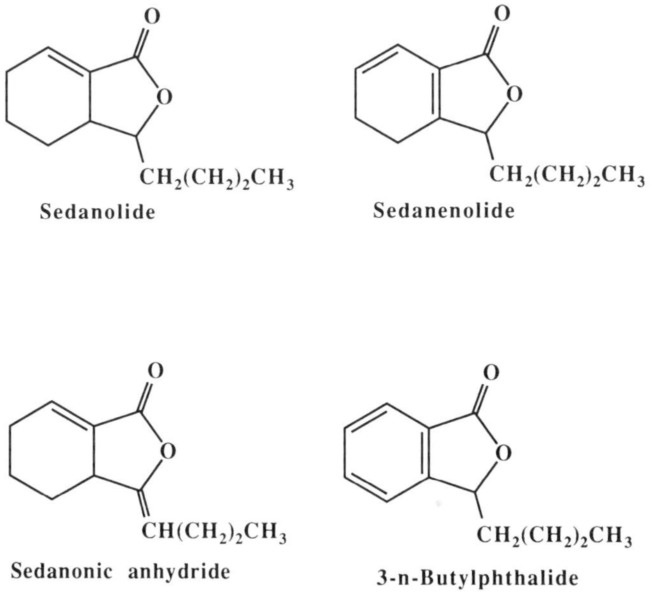

O
O
$CH_2(CH_2)_2CH_3$
Sedanolide

O
O
$CH_2(CH_2)_2CH_3$
Sedanenolide

O
O
$CH(CH_2)_2CH_3$
Sedanonic anhydride

O
O
$CH_2(CH_2)_2CH_3$
3-n-Butylphthalide

Figure 5.14 Structures of phthalides.

3. Licorice

Glycyrrhizic acid (Figure 5.15) is about 5–10% of the weight of the root of the licorice plant (*Glycyrrhize glabra L.*). Consumption of large amounts of licorice candy (100 g/day) over an extended period has led to severe hypertension, sodium retention, and heart enlargement in people. These symptoms apparently have as their basis a corticosterone-like activity in which sodium and water are retained and potassium is depleted. Severe losses of potassium resulting eventually in extreme weakness and ventricular fibrillation were reported in a woman who habitually ate nearly 2 kg of licorice candy per week.

4. Nutmeg

Nutmeg and its close relative, mace, have been used extensively in folk medicine for a wide range of ailments, including digestive disorders, rheumatism, cholera, and flatulence. There have also been a number of reports of nutmeg poisoning due to its use as an intoxicant. Nutmeg apparently acts as an intoxicant through its depressor effect on the central nervous system. Reactions to nutmeg vary from no effects to full-blown hallucinogenic experiences like those caused by hashish or LSD. Distortions of time and space with feelings of unreality have been reported. Effects of a single dose of approximately 20 g of whole nutmeg are reported to subside within 12–48 hr. Continued use of moderate doses

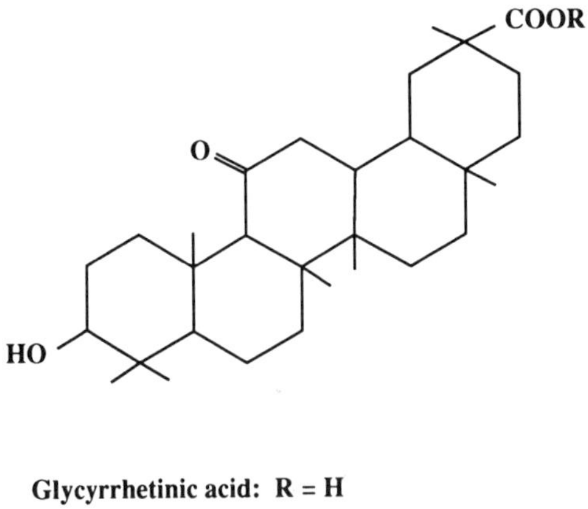

Glycyrrhetinic acid: R = H

Glycyrrhizic acid: R = Glucuronyl glucuronic acid

Figure 5.15 Structures of glycyrrhetinic acid and glycyrrhizic acid.

of nutmeg can result in liver damage and death. Side effects of even moderate doses of nutmeg include headache, cramps, and nausea. An active ingredient of nutmeg appears to be myristicin, which comprises approximately 4% of the oil. Myristicin (Figure 5.16) has also been identified in black pepper, parsley, celery, dill, and members of the carrot family. Pure myristicin is not as potent as whole nutmeg. Thus, it appears that other substances in addition to myristicin may be responsible for the psychoactive properties of this spice.

5. *Sassafras*

The essential oil of the root bark of the sassafras tree (*Sassafras albidum*) was used until 1960 in the United States as a flavor component of root beer. Teas prepared from the root bark are still apparently popular as tonics and for a variety of remedies in folk medicine. Results of a series of studies by the FDA showed that safrole, which comprises about 80% of the oil of sassafras, is a hepatocarcinogen in rats and mice. Administration of 0.04–1.0% of safrole in the diet of male and female rats for 150 days to 2 years produced hepatic cancers. As a result of these findings, safrole is no longer allowed as a food additive in the United States. The FDA also revised the banned substances listing of safrole specifically to ban sassafras bark, which is used primarily in the preparation of sassafras tea. Safrole is a component of many essential oils such as star anise and camphor oil. It also occurs in smaller quantities in mace, nutmeg, Japanese wild ginger, California bay laurel, and cinnamon leaf oil.

Safrole is related chemically to other substances found in spices. For example, β-asarone is a principal component of calamus oil (derived from the roots of *Acorus calamus*). The amount of β-asarone in the oil depends

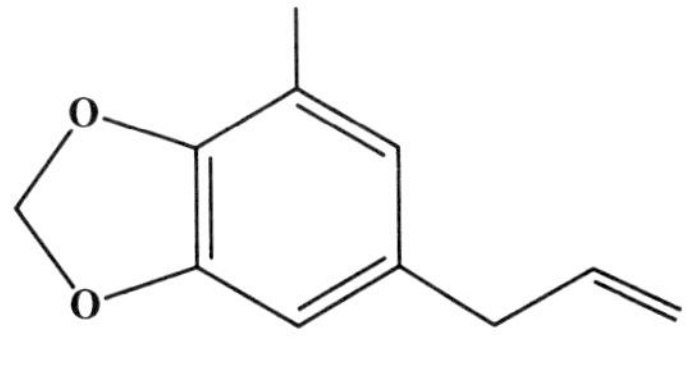

R
O
O

Myristicin: R = OCH_3

Safrole: R = H

Figure 5.16 Structures of myriscin and safrole.

on the variety of plant. The oil was formerly used in the preparation of vermouth and other flavored wines; however, β-asarone is no longer used legally in the United States because it was found to cause malignant tumors in the small intestine of rats fed on high doses. A similar substance is estragole, which is a component of tarragon oil, produced from *Artemisia dracunculus* and used as a flavor. Estragole causes liver cancer in young male mice.

Safrole provides an example of certain substances that are metabolically converted to the active carcinogenic forms. An extensive series of studies by Elizabeth and James Miller and their co-workers at the University of Wisconsin have demonstrated that safrole is metabolized in the rat and mouse to the corresponding benzylic alcohol (the proximate carcinogen), which, in turn, may be activated to the acetate or sulfate, the ultimate carcinogens (Figure 5.17). Nucleophilic attack on the double bond of the ultimate carcinogen by DNA may result in a heritable change in genetic material (a mutation). Subsequent expression of this altered genome may produce cancer. Because of the chemical similarities of

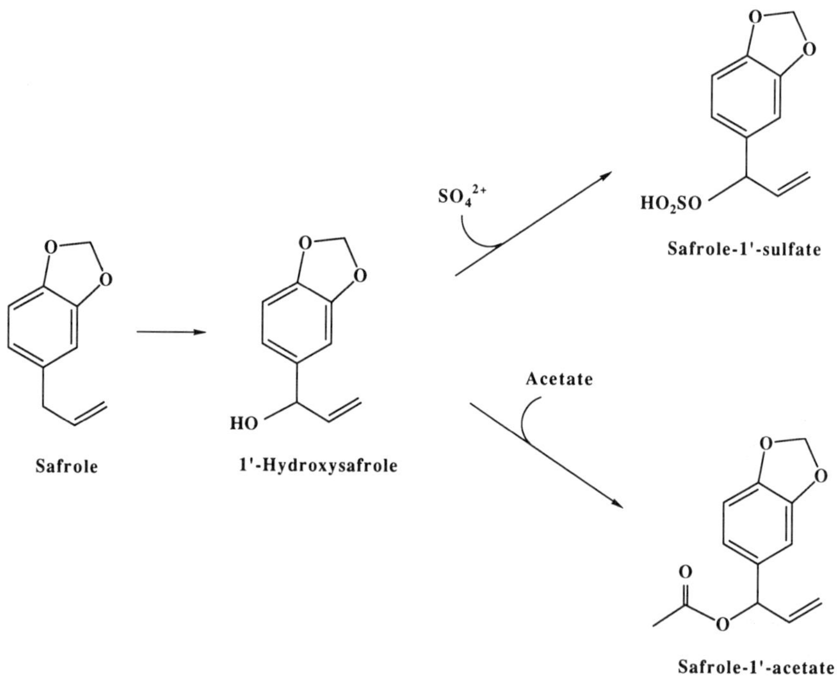

Figure 5.17 Metabolic pathways of safrole.

safrole, estragole, and β-asarone, it is likely that they are activated by similar processes.

E. Phytoalexins

Phytoalexins are antibiotics produced by a plant in response to environmental stresses. Various invading organisms such as bacteria, viruses, fungi, and nematodes will induce the production of phytoalexins in plants. In addition, exposure to cold, ultraviolet light, physical damage, and certain chemical compounds such as metal salts, polyamines, and certain pesticides can elicit the production of phytoalexins. Because phytoalexins are produced in response to such a broad range of agents that are potentially toxic to the plant, they are called stress metabolites. The classic example of phytoalexin production occurs in potatoes inoculated with the blight fungus, *Phytophthora infestans*. When inoculated into the potato, certain strains of this fungus will initially grow rapidly, followed by a gradual slowing of growth. If an extract of the infected material is placed in contact with a pure culture of the same fungus, the fungus will not grow. This phenomenon has been observed in many other plants such as peas, green beans, broad beans, soybeans, carrots, and sugar beets in response to infection by fungi. It appears that certain polysaccharide components of the cell wall of many fungi elicit this response.

The chemical composition of phytoalexins in general indicates that they are produced by modification of the plant's normal metabolism. Certain representatives of the widely occurring isoflavonoid and terpene classes of natural products are often responsible for the phytoalexin activity of injured plants (Figures 5.18, 19, and 20).

Quantities of phytoalexin produced by a plant can be quite significant. For example, soybeans infected with the fungus *Phytophthera megasperma* produce a phytoalexin known as glyceolin, which can accumu-

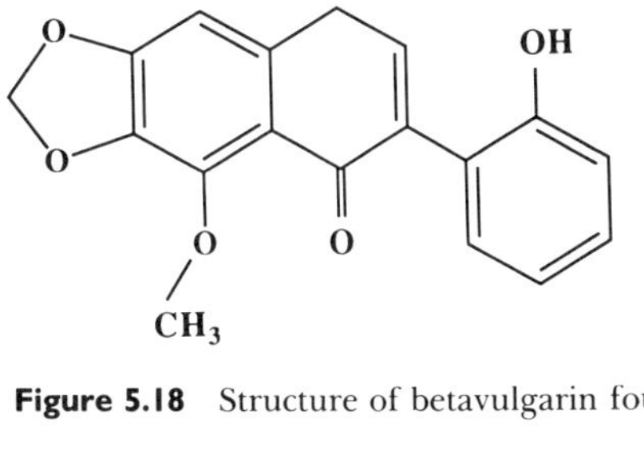

Figure 5.18 Structure of betavulgarin found in beets.

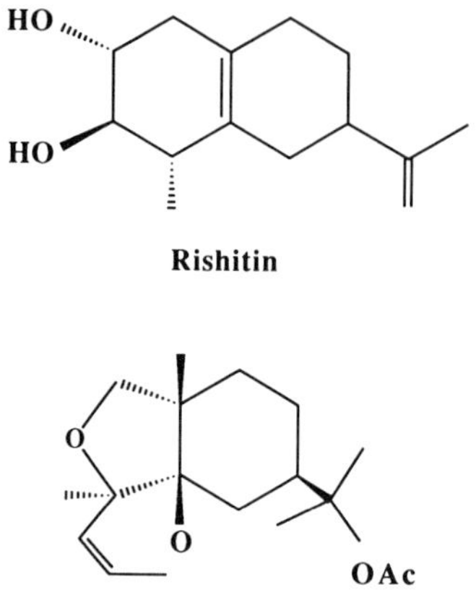

HO
HO
Rishitin

O
O
OAc
Phytuberin

Figure 5.19 Toxic substances found in potatoes.

late over a period of days from undetectable levels to more than 10% of the dry weight of the infected tissue.

In general, the toxicological aspects of phytoalexins have received little attention, but phytoalexins from partially rotted sweet potatoes have been studied in some detail. Consumption of sweet potatoes has been known to produce severe respiratory distress, pulmonary edema, congestion, and death in cattle. The sweet potatoes involved contained several toxic terpene substances (Figure 5.21). Two of the compounds, ipomeamarone and ipomeamaronol, cause liver degeneration in experimental animals (LD_{50} 230 mg/kg). Lung edema factors have also been isolated from the infected sweet potato tuber. The substances (Figure 5.22), known as 4-ipomeanol (LD_{50} 38 mg/kg), 1-ipomeanol (LD_{50} 79 mg/kg), ipomeanine (LD_{50} 26 mg/kg), and 1,4-ipomeadiol (LD_{50} 104 mg/kg), all produce an acute toxic response in mice that is indistinguishable from

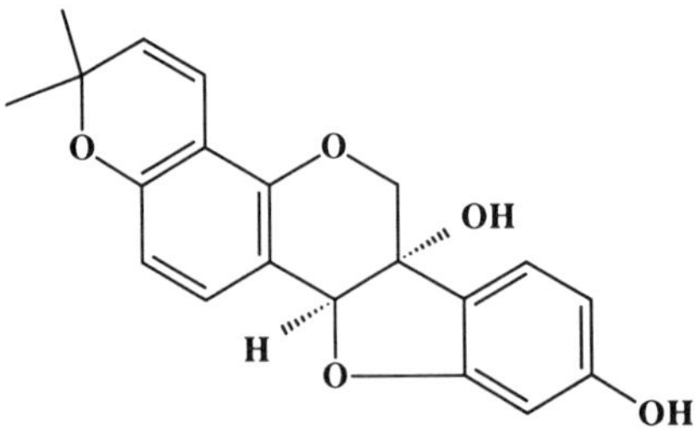

O
O
OH
H
O
OH

Figure 5.20 Structures of glyceolin found in soybeans.

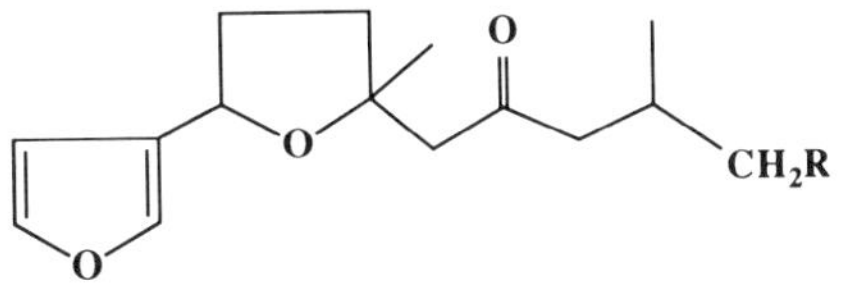

Ipomeamarone: R = H

Ipomeamaronol: R = OH

Figure 5.21 Structures of ipomeamarone and its alcohol.

the acute response produced by the administration of the crude sweet potato extract.

These toxic terpenes can occur in only slightly damaged sweet potatoes used as human food. The presence of these substances is always associated with darkening of the sweet potatoes. Ipomeamarone was shown in one study to be present in commercially available sweet potatoes at levels ranging from 0.1 to 7.8 mg/g sweet potato. Conflicting reports have appeared concerning stability of these toxic terpenes under normal cooking conditions. However, it appears that under conditions commonly employed in microwave cooking or baking, the concentration of iopmeamarone in sweet potatoes is reduced by 80–90%.

The phenomenon of toxic phytoalexin production must be considered in the debate over the use of pesticides. While pesticides have been used effectively to increase crop yield, their use has many drawbacks, including the nonspecific nature of their toxicity and their persistence in the environment. Plant breeders have been working, with some success,

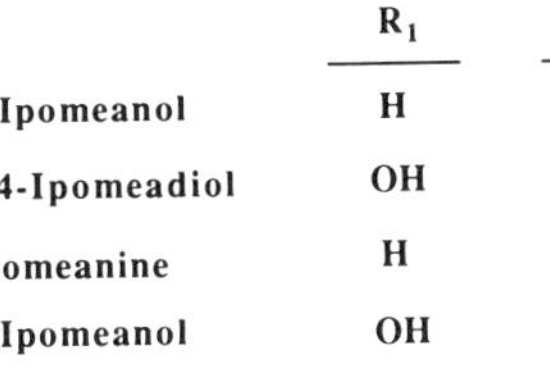

	R_1	R_2
4-Ipomeanol	H	OH
1,4-Ipomeadiol	OH	OH
Ipomeanine	H	O
1-Ipomeanol	OH	H

Figure 5.22 Toxic substances found in sweet potatoes.

to produce varieties of plants that are less dependent on pesticide use. However, this increased resistance of the various crops may result from high levels of phytoalexins. Until other means of pest control have been developed, it appears that the use of well-designed pesticides whose chemical, environmental, and toxic properties are already known may be preferable to developing new varieties of resistant crops with phytoalexins of unknown nature.

Suggestions for Further Reading

1. Delange, F., Iteke, F. B., and Ermans, A. M. (eds.) (1982). "Nutritional Factors Involved in the Goitrogenic Action of Cassava." International Development Research Centre, Ottawa.
2. Gaitan, E. (1989). "Environmental Goitrogenesis." CRC Press, Boca Raton, Florida.
3. Jadhav, S. J., Sharma, R. P., and Salunkhe, D. K. (1981). Naturally occurring toxic alkaloids in foods. *CRC Crit. Rev. Toxicol.* **9,** 21.
4. Liener, I. E. (ed.) (1980). "Toxic Constituents of Plant Foodstuffs," 2nd Ed. Academic Press, New York.
5. National Research Council (1973). "Toxicants Occurring Naturally in Foods," 2nd Ed. National Academy of Sciences, Washington, D.C.
6. Parker, A. J., Mehta, T., Zarghami, N. S., Cusick, P. K., and Haskell, B. E. (1979). Acute neurotoxicity of *Lathyrus sativus* neurotoxin, L-3-oxalylamino-2-aminopropionic acid, in the squirrel monkey. *Toxicol. Appl. Pharmacol.* **47,** 135.
7. Vennesland, B., Castric, P. A., Conn, E. E., Solomonson, L. P., Volini, M., and Westley, J. (1982). Cyanide metabolism. *Fed. Proc.* **41,** 2639.
8. Wargovich, M. J. (1987). Diallyl sulfide, a flavor component of garlic (*Allium sativum*), inhibits dimethylhydrazine-induced colon cancer. *Carcinogenesis* **8,** 487.
9. Watson, D. H. (ed.) (1987). "Natural Toxicants in Food: Progress and Prospects." VCH Publishers, New York.
10. Bailey, J. A., and Mansfield, J. W. (eds.) (1982). "Phytoalexins." Wiley, New York.
11. Grisebach, H. and Ebel, J. (1978). Phytoalexins, chemical defense substances of higher plants? *Angew. Chem. Int. Ed. Engl.* **17,** 635.

CHAPTER 6

Fungal Toxins Occurring in Foods

I. Mycotoxins

Fungi produce a multitude of substances of wide-ranging chemical structure and biological activity. Certain fungal metabolites are highly desired components in some foods such as cheese, while other metabolites are important antibiotics—penicillin, for instance. However, some fungi can produce substances that are potent acute toxins or carcinogens to both animals and humans. These toxic agents are generally called mycotoxins, a term usually reserved for toxins produced by filamentous fungi. The diseases these fungi cause are mycotoxicoses; their impact on domestic animals in terms of decreased growth rate, abnormal reproduction, disease, and early death has been known for centuries. The impact of these fungi in human illness has also been recognized for centuries, but their role as possible human carcinogens has been the subject of intensive study only since the early 1960s.

A. Ergotism

An association between the consumption of certain grains and human diseases was made early in history. Sacred writings of India (300–400 B.C.) refer to noxious grasses that caused pregnant women to abort or die in childbirth. Julius Caesar, in the first century B.C., is reported to have identified spoiled grain as the cause of certain epidemics that continued to occur regularly up to the Middle Ages in Europe.

By the middle of the 17th century, a cause and effect relationship was established between the consumption of grain contaminated with the fungus *Claviceps prupurea* (ergot) and disease. Under conditions of adequate moisture and warmth, the fungus invades individual grain kernels and form a sclerotium. The sclerotium, a lightly curved, black to purple body up to 6 cm long, is the resting stage of *Claviceps* and can remain viable under dry conditions and germinate when moistened. Today it is established that the growth of as many as 50 species of *Claviceps* on various food and feed crops in the grass family is associated with ergotism, the disease syndrome produced by ergot.

Gangrenous-type ergot poisoning may include severe pain, a burnt appearance of the affected limbs, and an inflammation of the extremities, which then turn black and, in severe cases, separate from the body. Because of the burnt appearance symptom, ergotism was called "holy fire" or "St. Anthony's Fire" in the Middle Ages from the belief that St. Anthony offered relief to those afflicted with the disease. A second type of ergotism that occurs under certain conditions is known as convulsive ergotism; it is characterized by neurological disorders such as numbness, blindness, paralysis, and convulsions.

The physiological basis of the gangrenous type of ergotism is the constriction of blood vessels. This activity has been exploited for centuries by the use of low doses of ergot to stop hemorrhage at childbirth. The blood vessel constriction results from a general stimulation of smooth muscles that is due to the direct effect on the muscle by ergot without the intervention of chemical or nervous mediators.

Ergot has also been used to induce uterine contraction during pregnancy. However, since uterine muscle is generally no more sensitive than other smooth muscle to the constrictive effects of ergot, a dangerously high dose must be used to induce uterine contraction in early pregnancy. However, uterine muscle becomes sensitive in the advanced stages of pregnancy and responds to much lower doses than the other smooth muscles during this period. Components of ergot are also used today as medications for certain complications during pregnancy.

The physiological basis for the selective occurrence of convulsive ergotism is poorly understood. Several hypotheses have been proposed, however, including the involvement of nutritional status of the afflicted individual, biosynthetic variability of the ergot fungus, genetic differences in susceptibility to ergot, and the possibility that another fungus may be parasitizing the ergot and introducing neurologically active substances. Resolution of these various possibilities requires further extensive research.

The principal pharmacologically active substances of ergot are a series of alkaloid derivatives that have lysergic acid as a part of their basic structure (Figure 6.1). Most important of the ergot alkaloids are ergotamine, ergonovine, and ergotoxin. Ergotamine was first isolated by Stowell in 1918 and is the first pure ergot alkaloid to find widespread medical application. Ergotamine tartrate is used almost exclusively in the treatment of migraine and other vascular headaches. Its mode of action is believed to involve vasoconstriction. Although the substance is very

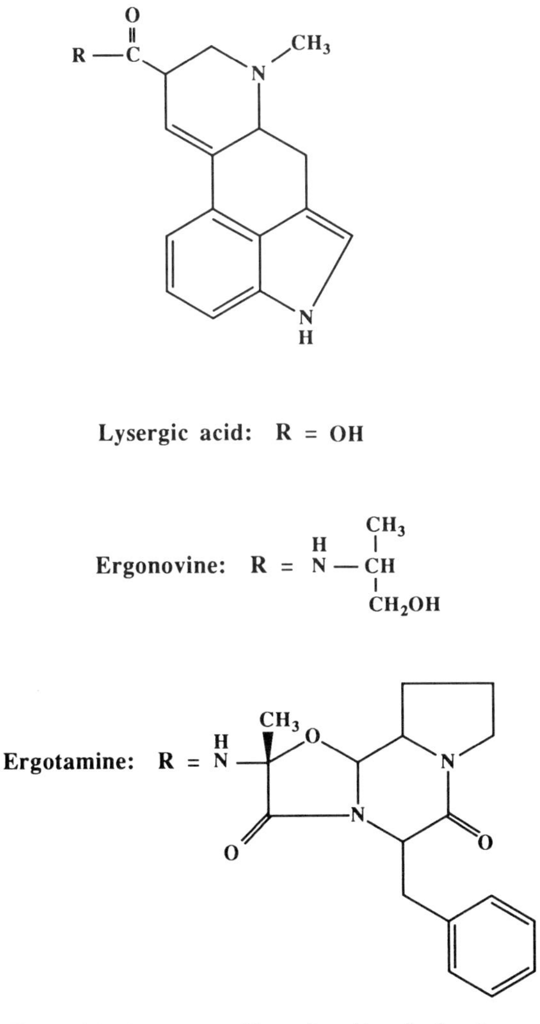

Lysergic acid: R = OH

Ergonovine: R = NH—CH(CH_3)CH_2OH

Ergotamine: R =

Figure 6.1 Structures of lysergic acid and related compounds.

effective against migraines, it is not suitable for long-term prophylactic use because of serious adverse effects such as severe vasoconstriction, resulting in dry gangrene of the extremities. Ergotamine is thought to be one of the substances primarily responsible for the characteristic gangrenous effect observed in ergot poisoning.

Ergonovine was first isolated in 1935 and found to be a potent inducer of uterine constriction. Ergonovine also causes significant vasoconstriction but does not exhibit the adrenergic blocking action of ergotamine. Ergonovine and a derivative, methyl ergonovine, are used in obstetrics in the third stage of labor, principally to decrease postpartum bleeding.

Ergotoxin is a crystalline mixture of ergocristine, ergokryptine, and ergocornine, all of which are similar in structure to ergotamine. The crystalline form of ergotoxin was first isolated from ergot in 1906. The ergotoxin group, like ergotamine, affects smooth muscle action and can block norepinephrine and epinephrine. A hydrogenated preparation of ergotoxin is useful in the treatment of peripheral and cerebral vascular disorders and essential hypertension. Synthetic amide derivatives of lysergic acid, including LDS, are highly potent hallucinogens in humans and as such are under intensive, continuing study.

B. Alimentary Toxic Aleukia

Alimentary toxic aleukia (ATA), or septic angina, is another mycotoxicosis that has caused great human suffering. ATA has been reported from time to time, primarily in Russia since the 19th century. Outbreaks were recorded in 1913, 1932, and toward the end of World War II. Russian accounts of symptoms of the disease include fever; hemorrhagic rash; bleeding in the nose, throat, and gums; necrotic angina; extreme leukopenia; agranulocytosis; sepsis; and modification of the bone marrow. Outbreaks of the disease were generally sudden, and mortality rates were often in excess of 50% of those afflicted. Russian scientists have identified four stages of the disease. The symptoms of Stage 1 generally appear shortly after consumption of the toxic food; they include burning sensations in the mouth, throat, esophagus, and stomach. This may be followed by vomiting, diarrhea, and abdominal pain due to inflammation of the gastric and intestinal mucosae. Patients at this stage also experience headaches, dizziness, fatigue, tachycardia, salivation, and fever; additionally, the blood leukocyte count is reduced. The symptoms may last from 3 to 9 days and then subside, signalling the onset of Stage 2. With the reduction in the intensity of the symptoms from the first stage, the patient may feel well and be capable of normal activity. However, at this stage, destruction of the blood-cell forming system progresses and there is continued reduction in lymphocytes accompanied by anemia. The body's resistance to bacterial infection is reduced; general weakness, headache, and reduced blood pressure are apparent. The duration of this second stage may be several weeks to months. If consumption of toxic food is stopped at this point and the patient is hospitalized, chances of recovery are very good. However, continued consumption of toxic food will lead to the onset of Stage 3. Stage 3 is signalled by the appearance of hemorrhages on the skin and on the mucous membranes of the mouth and tongue as well as in the intestine and stomach. As the toxicosis progresses, the necrotic lesions proliferate along with an increased tendency for bacterial infection. Esophageal lesions often occur and the involvement of the epiglottis may cause laryngeal edema leading in many cases to strangulation. Destruction of the hematopoietic system continues at this stage. If the patient survives Stage 3 by, for example, blood transfusions and administration of antibiotics, Stage 4, or the period of convalescence, is begun. Stage 4 often requires several months for the complete recovery of the hematopoietic system.

After rejecting several theories concerning the cause of the disease, such as vitamin deficiencies or infections, investigators eventually discovered that the disease was caused by consumption of grain left in the fields over the winter. Examination of the fungal flora of wintered cereals implicated in outbreaks of ATA revealed a rich array of fungal species. Toxicities of purified fungi, determined by application of fungal extracts to the skin of rabbits, were then associated with toxicity of moldy cereals to people. The rabbit skin assay was used for identification of toxic fungal strains and for subsequent efforts to identify active substances.

Fungi of the genus *Fusarium* were shown to produce the highest number of toxic isolates in the rabbit skin assay. The species most often associated with ATA outbreaks were *Fusarium poae* and *Fusarium sporotrichoides* (also called *Fusarium tricinctum*), which are fairly common species of fungi that have the peculiar capability of producing toxic substances in increased amounts when grown under conditions that include a period of growth at temperatures near 0°C.

In early studies, attempts to define the systematic sequence of ATA toxicosis were complicated by the variability of the disease. This variability was found to be due to the quantity and toxicity of material ingested, as well as other factors such as the age and nutritional status of the affected individual.

Early efforts by Russian scientists to isolate toxic substances responsible for ATA resulted in the identification of two steroidal compounds, one called sporofusarin from *Fusarium sporotrichoides* and another called poaefusarin from *Fusarium poae* (Figure 6.2). Efforts in the United States and elsewhere to isolate these substances from toxic *Fusarium* species were

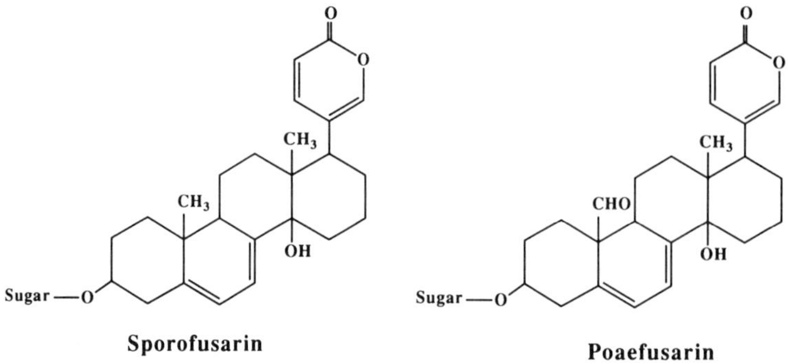

Sporofusarin

Poaefusarin

Figure 6.2 Structures of fusarins.

unsuccessful. Instead, substances of the trichothecin class were isolated (Figure 6.3). More recent efforts to confirm the toxicity of poaefusarin have shown that the sample contained enough trichothecins to account for the toxicity of the extract. In addition, examination of trichothecins produced by *F. poae* and *F. sporotrichoides* implicated in outbreaks of ATA established the production of toxic trichothecins by toxic isolates of these species. T-2 toxin (Figure 6.4) isolated from *F. sporotrichoides* and administered orally in gelatin capsules to cats produced all of the toxic symptoms characteristic of ATA. Removal of T-2 toxin from the *Fusarium* extract results in the loss of toxicity of the extract.

Although these studies clearly implicate T-2 toxin as a possible causative factor in the hemorrhagic lesions of ATA, results of other studies have suggested a more complicated etiology. For example, T-2 toxin administered orally to pigs and cats at a dose of 0.2 mg/kg body weight over a period of 78 days failed to induce clinical hemorrhagic syndromes. Chronic administration of T-2 toxin (20 ppm) to young mice showed that this species was susceptible both to the irritant and hematopoietic suppressive effects of dietary T-2 toxin, but that the suppression of hematopoiesis was transient and did not lead to hematopoietic failure.

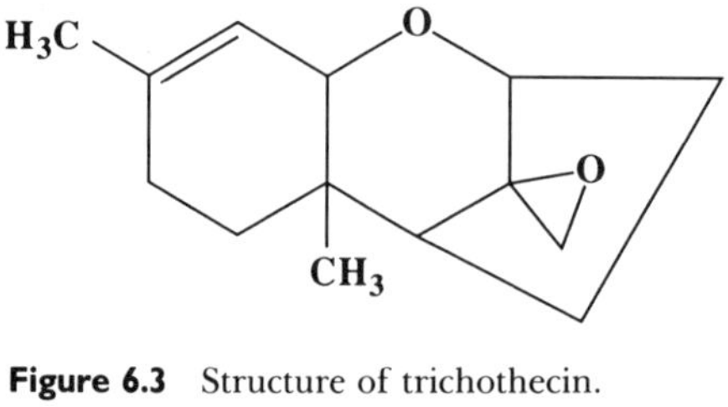

Figure 6.3 Structure of trichothecin.

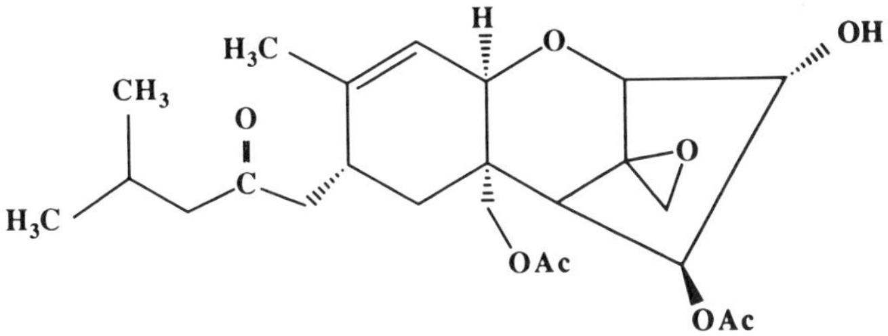

Figure 6.4 Structure of T-2 toxin.

The variability in response of various species to T-2 toxin may be due to several factors. These include

1. some species may be resistant to the suppressive effects of dietary T-2 toxin;
2. other toxins may be more important than T-2 toxin in the naturally occurring mycotoxicoses; and
3. dietary and other factors (including different mycotoxins) may increase the toxicity of T-2 toxin.

Thus, although tricothecenes such as T-2 toxin probably play a role in the etiology of ATA, the disease cannot be ascribed to a single substance and the complex interaction of trichothecenes with host variables must be unraveled before the etiology of ATA can be understood.

C. Aflatoxins

Moldy food has long been associated with various diseases in animals. These diseases were generally thought to be problems of livestock yield for farmers and the possible implications for human health were generally not considered. Various liver diseases, dubbed collectively "hepatitis–X" disease, were diagnosed by veterinarians in swine, cattle, and, in some cases, dogs. Improved methods of feed handling, production, and storage considerably reduced the occurrence of these types of diseases. It was not until 1960 that the human health implications of farm animal diseases began to be clearly recognized. At that time, over 100,000 young turkeys in England died of a disease that was dubbed "Turkey–X" disease. The disease was characterized by extensive necrosis of the liver in turkey poults. At the same time, attention was drawn to an increasing incidence of hepatic tumors in trout raised in hatcheries in the United

States. It was later shown that both the groundnuts (peanuts) used as a feed supplement for the turkeys and the cottonseed used as a feed supplement for the trout were contaminated by a series of compounds produced by a fungus known as *Aspergillus flavus*. These compounds, the aflatoxins, are not only potent acute toxins in several species, but are also some of the most potent hepatocarcinogens known.

Aflatoxins are a series of bisfuran polycyclic compounds (Figure 6.5). Based on their characteristic blue or green fluorescence under ultraviolet

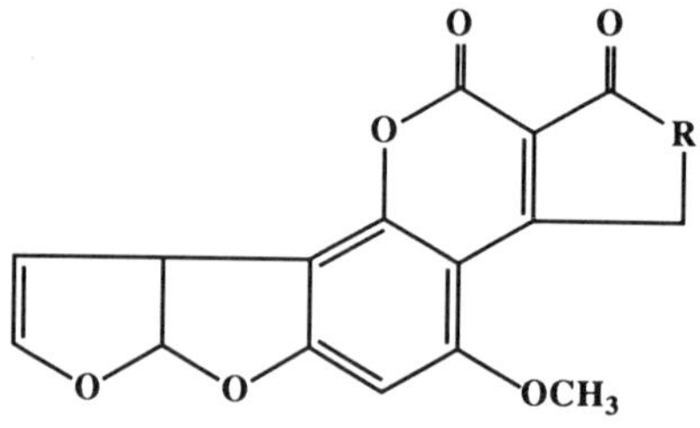

	R
Aflatoxin B_1	CH_2
Aflatoxin G_1	CH_2- O

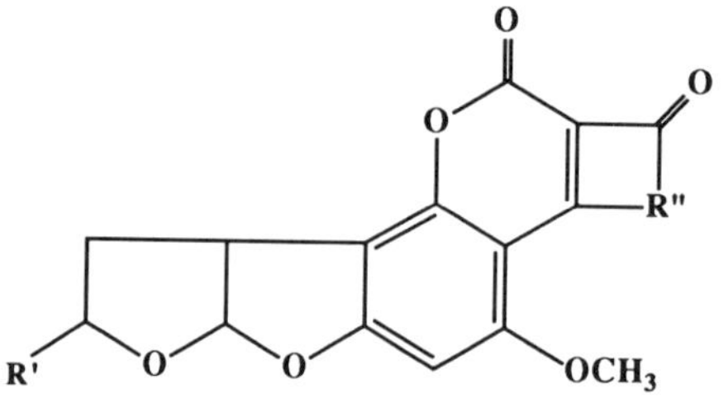

	R'	R"
Aflatoxin B_2	H	CH_2CH_2
Aflatoxin G_2	H	CH_2CH_2O
Aflatoxin B_2a	OH	CH_2CH_2
Aflatoxin G_2a	OH	CH_2CH_2O

Figure 6.5 Structures of aflatoxins.

light, these compounds were given the names aflatoxin B_1, B_2, G_1, and G_2, all of which are mold metabolites. Hydroxylated derivatives of aflatoxin B_2 and G_2 have also been isolated from mold and given the names aflatoxin B_{2a} and G_{2a}, respectively. The aflatoxins are lipid soluble and are not destroyed by most normal cooking conditions. They are also generally unstable when exposed to ultraviolet radiation.

1. Occurrence of Aspergillus flavus

Aspergillus flavus is a common constituent of the microflora in air and soil throughout the world. It causes deterioration of stored wheat, corn, rice, barley, bran, flour, and soybeans. In general, it does not invade the seeds of living wheat or intact peanuts. Growth occurs primarily when products are stored under conditions of relatively low moisture that eliminate the growth of competing species such as *Penicillium* and *Fusarium*.

With the development of sensitive assays for aflatoxins, many feed and food crops were analyzed for their presence. Assays conducted in the early 1960s in the United States showed that aflatoxins were present in the majority of peanuts and peanut meals produced in the United States and elsewhere. These assays also showed that roughly half of the peanut butter samples collected were contaminated with aflatoxins. Analyses of food samples collected from around the world, particularly from Africa and Asia, showed that aflatoxins could be detected in barley, cassava, corn, cottonseed, peas, millet, cowpeas, rice, sesame, sorghum, soybean, sweet potatoes, and wheat. Even dried spaghetti can contain aflatoxins. It is likely that aflatoxins are present in food and feed that are stored under conditions with enough moisture to allow the growth of *A. flavus* but not enough moisture to prevent the growth of other organisms.

2. Metabolism

Aflatoxin B_1 metabolism (Figure 6.6) has been studied in many species and under many different conditions. Aflatoxin B_1 is converted to at least seven metabolites, including a proposed unstable metabolite, the 8,9-epoxide, which is the so-called ultimate carcinogenic form (vide infra). Aflatoxin M_1 occurs in milk of cows fed on aflatoxin B_1-containing feeds. This metabolite is found in the liver, kidneys, and urine of sheep and in the livers of rats treated with aflatoxin B_1. The total conversion of aflatoxin B_1 to M_1 in cow's milk is estimated to be about 1%. In comparing carcinogenic activity in rats, aflatoxin M_1 is less than one-tenth as active

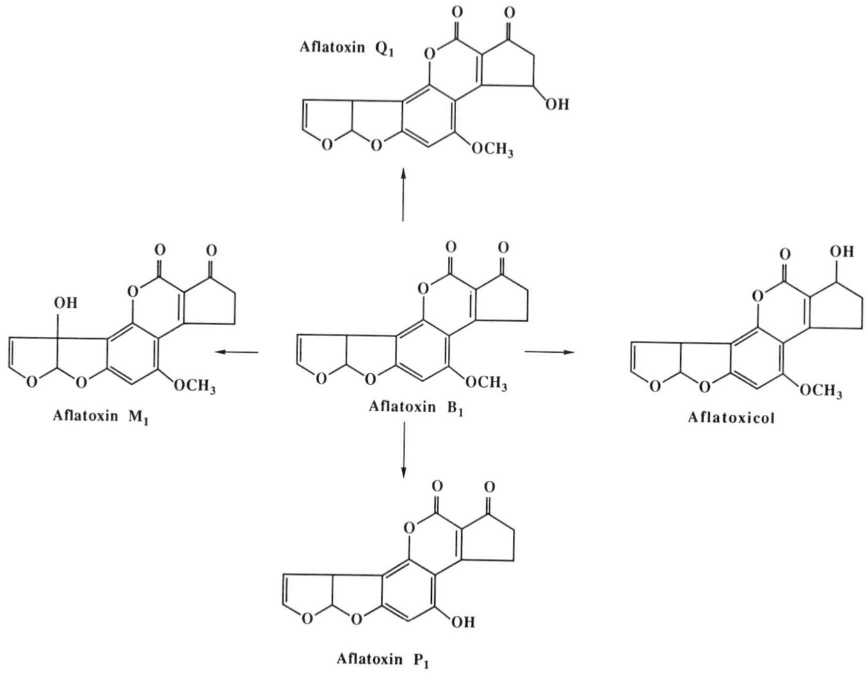

Aflatoxin Q_1

Aflatoxin M_1

Aflatoxin B_1

Aflatoxicol

Aflatoxin P_1

Figure 6.6 Metabolic pathways of aflatoxins.

as aflatoxin B_1. However, the acute toxicities of these substances are roughly similar. Aflatoxin M_1 generally comprises less than 2% of the total aflatoxin metabolites in the body.

Aflatoxicol, a reduction product of aflatoxin B_1, has roughly one-twentieth the acute toxicity of aflatoxin B_1 in the duckling bioassay but it has about one-fifth the mutagenic activity of aflatoxin B_1 in the Ames assay and roughly half the carcinogenic activity in trout. *In vivo,* it is readily oxidized to aflatoxin B_1 and may also serve as a reservoir for aflatoxin B_1. However, since the rate of aflatoxicol production in various test organisms is not consistently related to susceptibility to aflatoxin poisoning, its role in aflatoxicosis is unclear.

Two other major metabolites of aflatoxin B_1 are aflatoxins P_1 and Q_1. These substances have much lower acute toxicity than does aflatoxin B_1. Aflatoxin Q_1 is nontumorgenic in trout.

Evidence for the production of aflatoxin B_1-8,9-epoxide so far has been indirect but nevertheless substantial. Results of metabolic studies have shown that under certain circumstances an aflatoxin B_1-8,9-dihydro-8,9-diol can be isolated. In addition, an aflatoxin B_1 derivative

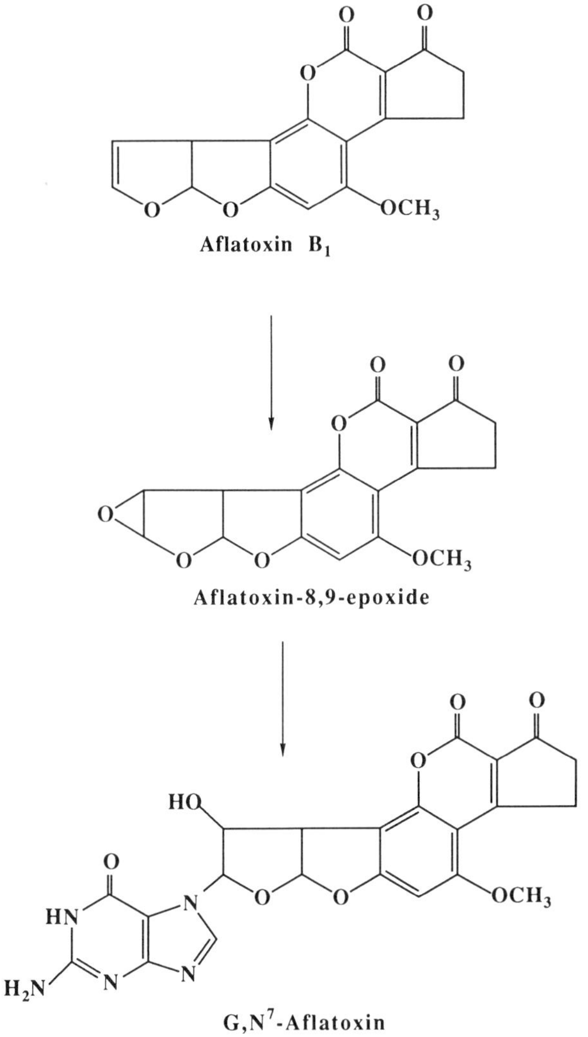

Aflatoxin B_1

Aflatoxin-8,9-epoxide

G,N^7-Aflatoxin

Figure 6.7 Formation of aflatoxin epoxide and guanine adduct.

has been isolated which is a likely product of binding of aflatoxin B_1-8,9-epoxide to guanine residues of nucleic acids (Figure 6.7).

3. Toxicities

Ducklings are the most sensitive species to the acute toxic effects of aflatoxins. The toxic potencies of aflatoxin B_1 in this assay are indicated in Table 6.1. Trout is also a sensitive species to the acute effects of

TABLE 6.1
Lethality of Single Doses (PO) of Alflatoxin B_1

Animal	Age	Sex	LD_{50} (mg/kg)
Duckling	1 day	M	0.37
Rat	1 day	M–F	1.0
Rat	21 days	M	5.5
Rat	21 days	F	7.4
Hamster	30 days	M	10.2

aflatoxins, whereas rats—and in particular, female rats—are relatively insensitive to the actue effects. Prominent acute effects in rats include hepatic lesions with edema, biliary proliferation, and parenchymal cell necrosis. In rhesus monkeys, aflatoxin treatment commonly results in fatty infiltration and biliary proliferation with portal fibrosis. There is considerable species variation in acute and chronic effects of aflatoxins. With regard to the chronic effects of aflatoxins, a high percentage of tumor induction was seen in male Fisher rats fed 2 ppm of aflatoxin B_1, while no tumor induction was seen in male albino mice fed aflatoxin B_1 at the same level. Sensitive species such as rats and trout show significant tumorigenesis when aflatoxin B_1 is fed at levels less than 100 ppb.

With the advent of sensitive analytical techniques for measuring aflatoxin levels in various crops and with a realization of the highly hazardous nature of these substances, the FDA has set limits on aflatoxin levels in food and feeds. Currently, the action limit for aflatoxins in milk is 0.5 ppb and in most foods it is 20 ppb. The maximum allowable limit for aflatoxins in animal feed is set at 100 ppb. Under these guidelines, millions of dollars worth of contaminated food and feed products have been seized by the FDA.

4. *Detoxification*

Many methods have been used in an effort to detoxify contaminated feeds. Physical separation of obviously contaminated materials has proven successful in controlling aflatoxin contamination in peanuts. *Aspergillus flavus* and several other fungi emit a bright yellow-green fluorescence under ultraviolet light. This telltale signal of fungal contamination has been useful in the physical separation of contaminated peanuts and corn as well as a few other crop samples.

Heat treatment of contaminated crops has also been used to detoxify food or feed material. Generally, under dry conditions the aflatoxins are quite heat stable. However, normal roasting conditions reduce the aflatoxin B_1 content in peanuts by 80% after half an hour. Heating under conditions similar to the moist conditions used for autoclaving are much more effective in reducing aflatoxin content than dry heating. This method has met with limited use, however. Several methods of solvent extraction have been employed with limited success. These methods are quite costly and time consuming and toxic components are not totally removed. In addition, essential nutrients may be extracted from the food or feed.

Several chemicals (such as hydrogen peroxide, ozone, and chlorine) have been used to destroy aflatoxins. These substances react readily with aflatoxins in foods as well as with many desired substances, including vitamins. The efficacy of these reagents in producing nontoxic yet nutritious material has not been established.

A more useful method of chemical detoxification of contaminated feed is treatment with ammonia. The use of ammonia to detoxify corn meal and cottonseed meal increases the nutritional value of the feed. The detoxified feed supports the growth of trout, cows, and other animals without apparent ill effects. An ammoniation process developed in Arizona involves placing a mixture of aqueous ammonia and cottonseed in large plastic bags commonly used for silage. The bags are sealed and allowed to stand in the sun for several weeks. The process has been shown to be effective in reducing the levels of aflatoxin in highly contaminated cottonseed (800 ppb) to less than the 100 ppb action levels set by the FDA.

5. General Considerations

Studies of the importance of aflatoxins in the etiology of human cancer have concentrated primarily on areas of Southeast Asia, China, and Africa where aflatoxin levels in the food are relatively high. Continuing analyses of the combined epidemiological data from several such studies indicate that high-level intake of aflatoxin in combination with such other diseases as hepatitis is associated with an increased rate of liver cancer. Whether aflatoxins by themselves are human hepatocarcinogens remains the subject of scientific controversy. Despite these uncertainties about the role of aflatoxins in human cancer, efforts to minimize human exposures continue. There are well-established methods of harvesting, drying, and storing crops that are effective in the control of fungal contamination and aflatoxin production. Efforts are ongoing to implement these techniques in areas of high aflatoxin contamination in the hope of reducing the incidence of liver cancer.

II. Other Mycotoxins

Following the dramatic discovery of the aflatoxins, many investigators initiated studies on other fungi that occur on food and feed. Many toxins have been isolated from other fungi but their effects are much less dramatic than those of the aflatoxins and they have not been as thoroughly studied. A general screening program with ducklings as the test organism showed that most of the strains of *Aspergillus ochraceous* were toxigenic. *Aspergillus ochraceus,* a mold similar to *A. flavus,* occurs widely in nature and is found in the soil and on decaying vegetation. Toxic substances isolated from *A. orchraceus* include ochratoxins A and B (Figure 6.8). *Aspergillus ochraceus* is a predominant fungus on red and black peppers and is found in stored cottonseed, citrus fruit, peanuts, and tobacco. The fungus has also been used in Japan to produce fermented fish, which is known as katsuo bushi. In albino rats, ochratoxin A has an LD_{50} of 20 mg/kg. It produces liver degeneration but it is apparently not carcinogenic. Ochratoxin B is much less toxic. The ochratoxins are hydrolyzed in the liver and secreted in the bile.

Rubratoxins (Figure 6.9) are acute toxins produced by *Penicillium rubrum* with apparently no carcinogenic effects. The LD_{50} of rubratoxin A is 6.6 mg/kg by intraperitoneal injection in rats. Administration of these toxins to animals causes extensive liver and kidney damage.

Considerable work has been done in Japan on the potential hazard of moldy or yellowed rice. Many fungi and many of their toxic metabolites have been isolated. Yellowed rice toxins are mentioned here because two

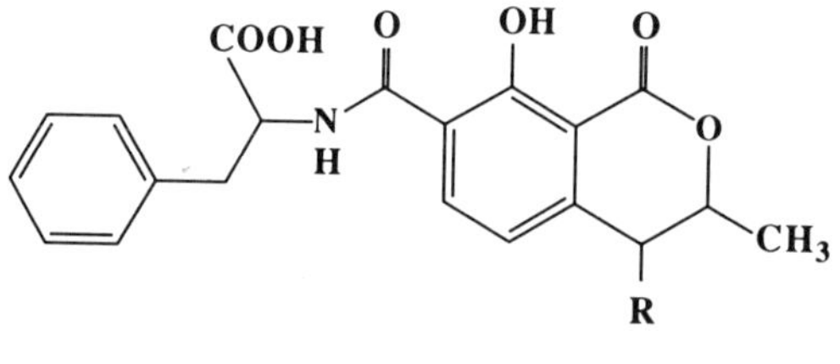

COOH O OH O
N O
H
CH_3
R

Ochratoxin A: R = Cl

Ochratoxin B: R = H

Figure 6.8 Structures of ochratoxins.

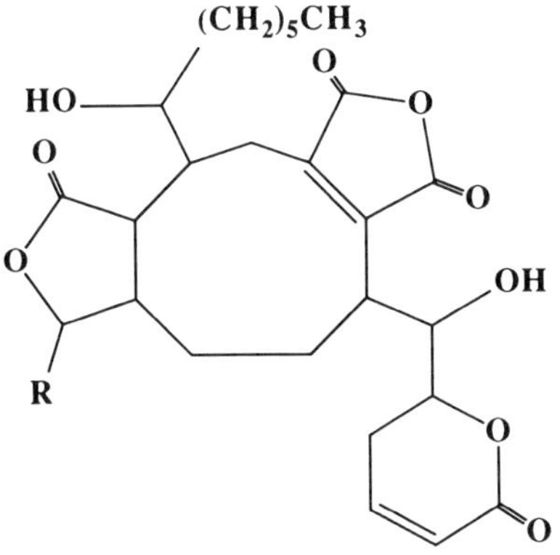

Rubratoxin A: R = OH

Rubratoxin B: R = O

Figure 6.9 Structures of rubratoxins.

implicated fungi, *Penicillium islandicum* and *Penicillium rugulosum,* are the first non-*Aspergillus* species identified which produce tumorigenic substances. Administration of approximately 200 g/day of rice infected with *Penicillium islandicum* for 1 week causes the death of laboratory animals from liver necrosis. In another study, a high percentage of animals developed liver tumors following 2 years of consuming a diet that contained a 0.05 g/day of moldy rice. Few malignant tumors were observed, however. Three of the active components in the yellowed rice are rugulosin, luteoskyrin, and islandicin (Figure 6.10). Liver necrosis is the primary cause of death in mice following treatment with rugulosin (LD_{50} = 83 mg/kg) and luteoskyrine (LD_{50} = 7 mg/kg). Prolonged feeding of luteoskyrine to mice at a relatively high dose (50 mg/kg) resulted in liver tumors. Islanditoxin, a highly toxic cyclic peptide produced by *P. islandicum,* causes severe liver damage, hemorrhage, and death in animals when administered in low oral doses (LD_{50}-7 mg/kg).

An estrogenic substance, zearalenone (Figure 6.11), is produced by the fungus *Fusarium roseum* and its sexual stage, *Gibberella zeae,* as well as by related fungi. Consumption of corn infected with these fungi causes loss of reproductive capacity and other estrogenic effects in pigs and other animals. Symptoms of zearalenone poisoning in young pigs include swelling and eversion of the vagina until in some cases the cervix is visible.

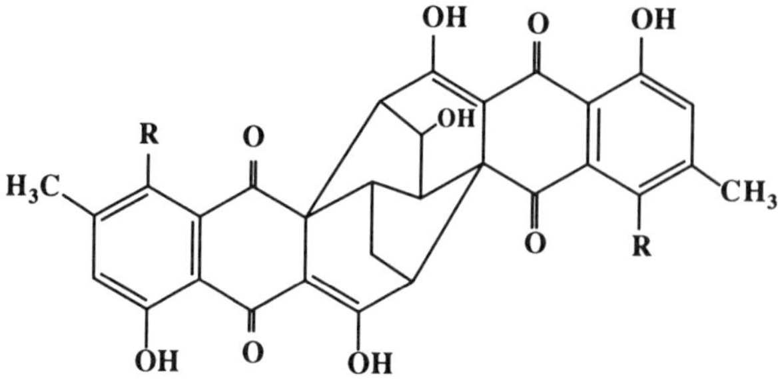

Rugulosin: R = H

Luteoskyrin: R = OH

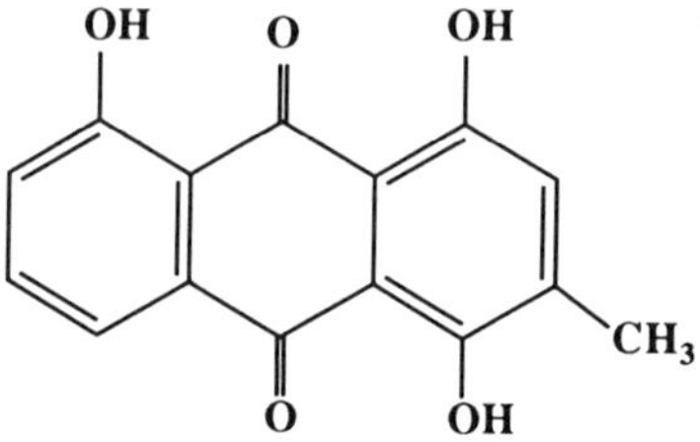

Islandicin

Figure 6.10 Structures of toxins isolated from yellow rice.

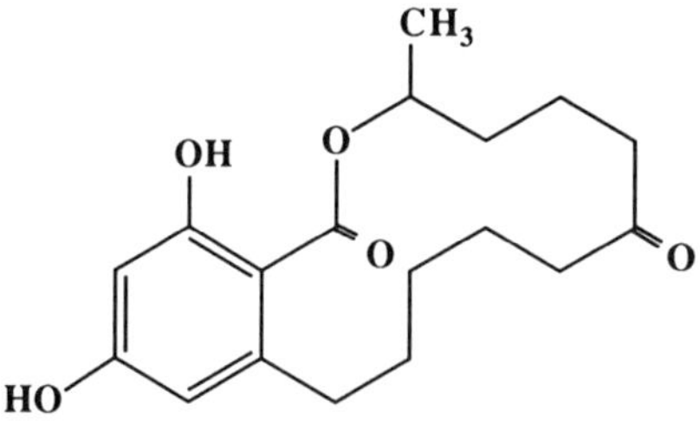

Figure 6.11 Structure of zearalenone.

III. Mushroom Fungal Toxins

Mushrooms are a delicacy to people the world over. A few species are grown commercially in the United States and are consumed in vast quantities with considerable enjoyment. But health problems can arise from the consumption of wild mushrooms. In the United States, only about 50 of the over 800 identified species are known to produce some toxic effects in people. In most cases, an unwary collector can consume a mildly toxic species of mushroom and most likely suffer only simple gastrointestinal upset that will soon pass. For various potentially toxic mushrooms, special cooking processes have been developed to render them edible. Only a few species are considered highly toxic or lethal if consumed. One genus in particular (*Amanita*) contains some of the most notorious as well as the best tasting mushroom species.

Amanita muscaria is a classic example of a psychoactive and toxic mushroom. This fleshy fungus grows throughout temperate areas of the world. It is not sought after as a food; instead, it has been used for many centuries as a hallucinogen. The pleasant effects of this mushroom and the reported slow degradation of the active principles combine to make *A. muscaria* a prized component of tribal and religious rituals in many parts of the world. Use of *A. muscaria* as a narcotic or intoxicant is well documented. Substances primarily responsible for the narcotic-intoxicant effect are a series of isoxazoles, such as muscimol (Figure 6.12), that comprise approximately 0.20% of the dry weight of *A. muscaria.* The neurological symptoms of individuals who have consumed *A. muscaria* vary, but they generally begin to occur 30–90 min following ingestion. A state resembling alcoholic intoxication is generally produced. Confusion, restlessness, visual disturbance, muscle spasms, and delirium may follow. Patients are reported to pass into a deep sleep following the excited period, and upon waking, they may have little or no memory of the experience. Ingestion of 15 mg of pure muscimol by a single individual

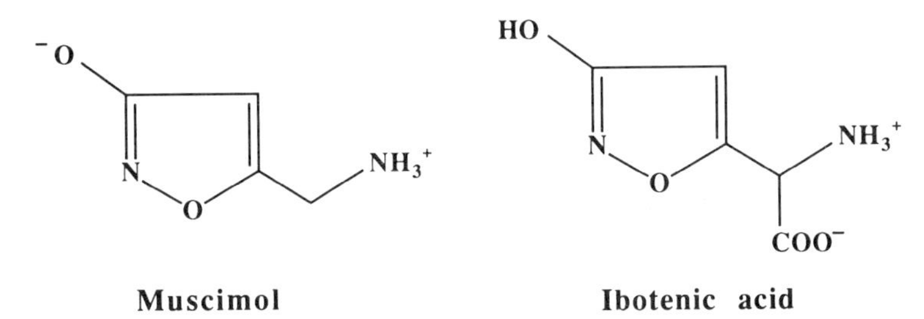

Figure 6.12 Structures of muscimol and ibotenic acid.

is reported to cause confusion, visual disturbance, illusions of color vision, fatigue, and sleep.

Ibotenic acid (Figure 6.12), another isoxazole present in the mushroom, is reported to produce no psychic stimulation. This compound induces lassitude and sleep that is followed by a migraine and a lesser and localized headache that lasts for weeks. The overall response in an individual is unpredictable since individual susceptibilities differ and since the levels of the isoxazole and muscarine vary in the mushroom due to environmental and genetic factors.

Amanita muscaria is known as fly agaric because it contains muscarine, the principal substance responsible for the fly-killing activity of *A. muscaria* and a few other mushrooms. Muscarine is a fairly simple compound (Figure 6.13) that in comparatively small doses (0.01 mg/kg) reduces blood pressure in cats. Muscarine acts like acetylcholine on the receptors of smooth muscles and glandular cells, the so-called muscarinic receptors.

The symptoms of muscarine poisoning appear within 30 min of ingestion. Symptoms include increased salivation, lachrymation, and perspiration followed by vomiting and diarrhea. Pulse is slow and irregular and breathing is asthmatic. Death is uncommon, and patients generally respond well to atropine sulfate. Severe cases of muscarine poisoning are rare. This indicates that the levels of muscarine relative to the levels of other substances that are causing the desired narcotic effect of the mushroom are generally quite low.

Amanita phalloides, also known as the death cap mushroom, is perhaps the most well-known toxic mushroom. This species is said to be responsible for 90–95% of all mushroom poisoning deaths in Europe. It has also been responsible for several deaths each year in the United States, where it was fairly rare until the early 1970s, when it apparently entered the western United States in a nursery specimen from Europe. The mushrooms, or fruiting bodies, of *A. phalloides* generally appear in the late summer or fall and can stand 8" tall. The color of the relatively large cap can range from greenish-brown to yellow. *Amanita phalloides*, because of its size and close similarity to other highly edible and sought-after species of *Amanita*, is often a prize find of avid mushroom hunters.

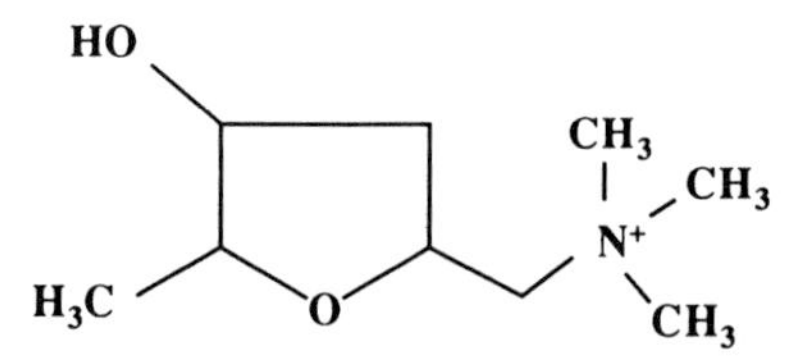

Figure 6.13 Structure of muscarine.

Amanita phalloides contains several cyclic peptides that account for the toxicity of the mushroom. The substances are of two types and have been called phalloidins and amanitins. The phalloidins are highly toxic in tissue cultures and when injected into test animals; however, they are weakly toxic when administered orally. The amanitins have LD_{50}'s in mice in the order of 0.1 mg/kg and are toxic when administered orally or intravenously. It has been hypothesized that the phalloidins are responsible for the initial gastrointestinal phase of poisoning, whereas the more toxic but slower acting amanitins are responsible for the later phase of toxicity which occurs after 3–5 days and affects the liver and kidneys.

The principal toxic component of *Amanita phalloides* is α-amanitin (Figure 6.14) which acts specifically to inhibit an enzyme, RNA polymerase, required to synthesize messenger RNA. The cellular effects of α-amanitin include disintegration of nucleoli in liver cells, which prevents ribosome synthesis and ultimately protein synthesis. Destruction of the convoluted tubule of the kidney is also caused by α-amanitin, which diminishes kidney's effectiveness in filtering toxic non-electrolytes from the blood.

The chemical structures of the amanitins and the phalloidins are complex indeed. The phalloidins and amanitins are cyclic peptides that contain seven and eight amino acids, respectively. There is evidence to suggest that these cyclic peptides are mere fragments of much more complex polysaccharide components. These large molecular-weight substances, which are called myriamanins, may be isolated by a mild solvent

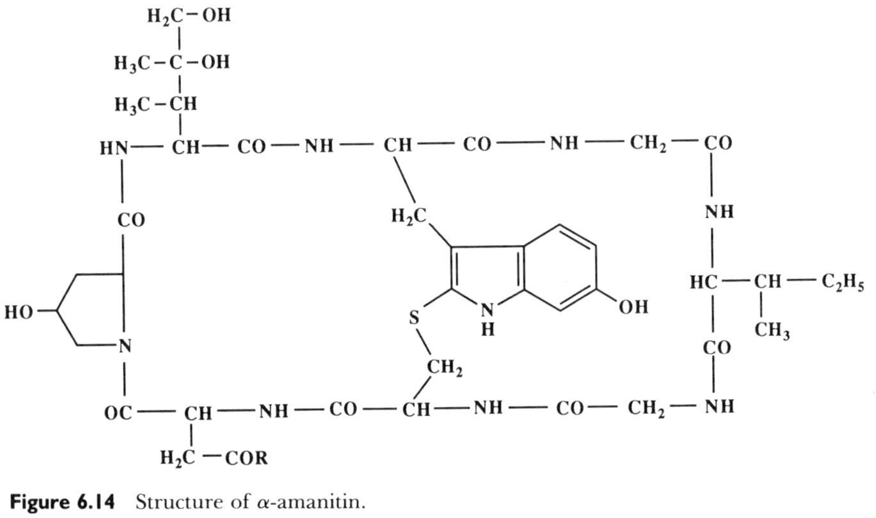

Figure 6.14 Structure of α-amanitin.

extraction of the mushrooms. Molecular masses as high as 60,000 Da have been assigned to some of these active components. The smaller cyclic peptides are obtained from these larger compounds by strong acid or alkaline treatment.

Toxic symptoms appear many hours following consumption of *A. phalloides.* Initial signs of toxicity are abdominal pain, diarrhea, and vomiting. If an adult has consumed at least two caps of the mushroom, death will occur from dehydration if the individual is not treated to restore proper electrolyte balance. Any individual who survives this stage of poisoning is still in jeopardy of succumbing to subsequent toxic effects. Death in most cases is due to extensive liver and kidney damage. Attempts to find antidotes for *Amanita* poisoning have been generally unsuccessful. However, a preparation of cytochrome c appears to be somewhat useful in treatment of toxic effects of α-amanitin. Results of experiments with mice have shown cytochrome c to be effective in improving survival of mice, even when the treatment was withheld for 8 hr following administration of the toxin. Although the mechanism of this protective effect has not been established, this treatment and others have been used successfully in cases of human poisoning. Human survival rates have increased in recent years to above 50% and are likely to increase further as our understanding of the basic enzymology of *Amanita* poisoning becomes more complete.

Suggestions for Further Reading

1. Bresinsky, A., and Besl, H. (1990). "A Colour Atlas of Poisonous Fungi: A Handbook for Pharmacists, Doctors, and Biologists." Woolfe, London.
2. Hathcock, J. N. (ed.) (1982–1989). "Nutritional Toxicology." Academic Press, New York.
3. Hayes, A. W. (1981). "Mycotoxin Teratogenicity and Mutagenicity." CRC Press, Boca Raton, Florida.
4. Kadis, S., and Ciegler, A., and Ajl, S. J. (eds.) (1972). "Microbial Toxins." Academic Press, New York.
5. Purchase, I. F. J. (ed.) (1974). "Mycotoxins." Elsevier, New York.
6. Rodericks, J. V. (ed.) (1976). "Mycotoxins and Other Fungal Related Food Problems." Advances in Chemistry Series 149. American Chemical Society, Washington, D.C.
7. Wogan, G. N. 1966. Chemical nature and biological effecs of the aflatoxins. *Bacterio Rev.* **30:**460.

CHAPTER 7

Food Contaminants from Industrial Wastes

Through industrial activities in the modern era, many potentially hazardous substances have been put into the environment through ignorance, accident, and irresponsibility. However, as knowledge of toxicology and analytical capabilities have improved, both a clearer understanding of the potential toxicity and an awareness of the health hazards caused by these contaminants have been gained. The most widely studied of these substances are lead, mercury, cadmium, polychlorinated biphenyls, and tetrachlorodibenzo-*p*-dioxin.

I. Chlorinated Hydrocarbons

A. Polychlorinated Biphenyls

Polychlorinated biphenyl (PCB) is a generic term used to describe a number of chlorinated derivatives of biphenyl (Figure 7.1). There are a total of 210 combinations possible, but there may be only 102 actually present. PCBs that are generally available commercially are a mixture of different substances that are sold in formulations varying by the percentage of chlorine in the substance. For example, in the United States, PCBs are sold by the trade name Aroclor, followed by different designations such as 1242, 1248, 1260. The last two digits of these designations indicate the percentage of chlorine in the preparation.

Not long after the first synthesis of PCBs, it became obvious that

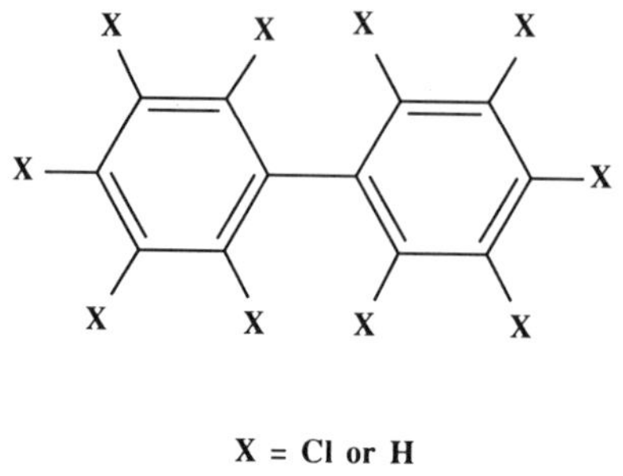

X = Cl or H

Figure 7.1 Structures of polychlorinated biphenyls.

these compounds were unusual organic molecules. They were found to have considerable resistance to acids, bases, water, high temperatures, and electrical currents. With the discovery of these properties, PCBs found widespread use in the 1930s as insulating fluids in electrical transformers and capacitors, as well as in hydraulic fluids where resistance to high temperatures was required.

1. Environmental Impact

Environmental contamination by PCBs received little attention until the 1960s. At that time the scientific community became concerned about the levels of chlorinated hydrocarbon pesticides such as DDT in food. PCBs, being close chemical relatives of DDT, began to show up as an unidentified contaminant of analytical samples. In many cases, PCBs were present in much higher quantities than was DDT. Subsequent concerted efforts to determine the levels of PCBs in foods indicated that the levels were highly dependent on the type of food analyzed.

Environmental impact of PCBs would be relatively small if the uses of these substances were restricted to the electrical components in which PCBs occur in sealed containers. However, because of the clear, oily, highly stable nature of these substances, they have been used extensively also in plasticizers, paints, lubricants, and insulating tapes. They have also found their way into fireproofing materials, inks, carbonless copy paper, and pesticide preparations.

Vast quantities of PCBs have been produced. It is estimated that by 1977, when production of PCBs in the United States was almost completely discontinued, over a billion pounds of these substances had been produced in the United States. Because of their high degree of stability, only about 600 million pounds of these substances are estimated to be degraded or destroyed, which leaves about 450 million pounds of discarded PCBs still present in some form in the environment. These figures represent only a part of the total quantity of PCBs in the world environment, since PCBs were produced by manufacturers in several other countries as well.

2. *Occurrence*

The same properties of high stability and lipid solubility that made PCBs highly sought after for industrial uses resulted in their bio-accumulation in the food chain. Market basket food analyses in 1971–1972 indicated PCB levels in foods available for general consumption always to be less than about 15 ppb except for certain food oils, which in some cases reached levels as high as 150 ppb. The highest levels of PCB contamination were found in fish from the Great Lakes. Chinook salmon from Lake Michigan contained levels of 10–24 ppm PCB. Lake trout from Lake Michigan contained levels of 8–21 ppm. As expected, other wildlife dependent on fish as part of their food also contained high levels of PCB. Analyses of dolphin tissue from locations near the coast of California indicated levels on the order of 150 ppm based on fat. Analyses of blubber from porpoises and whales from the East and West coasts of the United States indicated levels of 74 and 46 ppm. The accumulation of PCBs in birds was evident from analyses of eggs. Heron eggs from the Netherlands contained PCBs in the range of 34–74 ppm.

Massive surveys of PCB levels in human adipose tissue in the United States and surveys of PCBs in human milk showed levels generally in the range of about 0.1–3.0 ppm based on fat. These PCB levels in human tissues were dependent primarily on consumption of contaminated fish. Thus, consumption of fish from contaminated waters such as some of the Great Lakes was shown to be highly correlated with the level of PCBs found in human blood.

The revised permissible levels of PCB in food established by the FDA are 2 ppm in fish and shellfish, 1.5 ppm based on milk fat and dairy products, 3 ppm in poultry fat, and 0.3 ppm in eggs. Although the FDA has authority only over products shipped by interstate commerce, it has advised individual states where high levels of PCBs have been detected to consider establishing similar tolerances for PCB levels in their food products, especially fish. Several states have established these tolerances and in some cases this has meant the prohibition of commercial fishing in these areas.

3. In Vivo *Absorption and Metabolism*

The absorption and excretion characteristics of PCBs are as expected for stable fat-soluble substances. Thus, dietary PCBs are extensively absorbed from the gastrointestinal tract, with greater than 90% absorption common for most of these substances. The absorbed PCBs are stored primarily in adipose tissue with intermediate concentrations in the skin, adrenal glands, and aorta and the lowest concentrations in the blood. Concentrations decrease with time most rapidly from the blood and most slowly from the adipose tissue. The biologic half-life of PCBs is estimated to be 8 weeks in male rats and 12 weeks in female rats.

The metabolism of PCBs is also strongly influenced by the extent of chlorination. The biphenyl derivatives that contain less chlorine are metabolized and excreted more rapidly than the biphenyl derivatives with higher percentages of chlorine. The route of metabolism of PCBs is primarily by conversion to the corresponding phenols with loss of chlorine. The principal route of excretion of PCBs is through the feces with a relatively small percentage (less than 10%) showing up in the urine. This extensive elimination via the gastrointestinal tract, in spite of efficient absorption, suggests a major role for biliary excretion for PCBs. Excretion of PCBs via the milk in humans is generally minor in comparison to fecal and urinary excretion. However, the primary mode of excretion of PCBs in lactating cattle is via milk. Thus, cattle fed PCB-contaminated feed produce contaminated milk.

4. *Mode of Toxic Action and Toxicities*

The acute and chronic effects of PCBs have been studied extensively in several animal species including rabbits, mice, pigs, sheep, and monkeys. Chicks fed PCBs at 50 ppm in the diet exhibit symptoms of depressed weight gain, edema, gasping for breath, hyperparacardial fluid, internal hemorrhaging, depression of secondary sexual characteristics, and increased liver size. Pigs and sheep appear to be less sensitive to the toxic effects of PCBs than monkeys. In pigs, dietary PCBs at levels of 20 ppm during the normal period of growth before slaughter resulted only in reduced feed efficiency and reduced rate of weight gain. The pigs had gastric lesions along with an increased frequency of pneumonia. Sheep appeared to be unaffected by dietary PCBs.

Acute toxic effects produced in adult rhesus monkeys at PCB levels of 250–400 mg/kg body weight include the development of gastric mucosal hypertrophy and hyperplasia, generalized hair loss, edema, and acne. In one study, the acne, edema, and hair loss were still present 8 months after cessation of PCB administration, indicating a slow recovery from the toxic effects.

Adverse reproductive effects of PCBs have been observed in several other animal species. Chickens fed 50 ppm PCB produced chicks with leg, toe, and neck deformities. Also, eggs produced from the exposed hens showed a significant increase in the percentage of non-viable embryos. In rabbits, 25 mg/kg PCB in the diet for 21 days caused abortion in one out of four animals. Mice weaned on milk containing PCB produced litters of fewer pups. Prolonged ingestion of dietary PCB at 150 ppm reduced reproductive capacity of female rats in addition to reducing plasma hormone (progesterone) level.

In a study with female rhesus monkeys, relatively small doses (2.5–5.0 ppm) of PCBs in the diet resulted in symptoms of chloracne (severe acne-like skin eruptions) and edema. Menstrual cycles were changed, and problems of maintaining pregnancies occurred. Successful pregnancies produced infants of relatively low body weight. Fatty tissues of these infants contained PCBs at levels of approximately 25 ppm. Male rhesus monkeys receiving high doses of PCBs (5ppm) showed only minor symptoms of toxicity with no evidence of reproductive effects.

The liver appears to be uniquely sensitive to the effects of PCB. Increased liver weight, liver hypertrophy, proliferation of smooth endoplasmic reticulum, and an increase in microsomal enzyme activity characterize PCB effects in this organ. The activities and levels of certain cytochrome P450 enzymes increase dramatically following administration of PCBs, while the activity of glucose 6-phosphatase and the levels of vitamin A in the liver decrease dramatically.

PCBs may be involved in carcinogenesis in at least two ways. First, since many carcinogens require metabolic activation mediated by the cytochrome P450 enzyme system, PCBs may increase or decrease the carcinogenic potency of these compounds, depending on the role of specific metabolic processes in their conversion to active and inactive forms. Second, results of experiments with rats indicate that PCBs are themselves carcinogenic. In one experiment, long-term administration of PCBs (Aroclor 1260) at a level of 100 ppm to female rats resulted in liver tumors in 26 of 184 experimental animals administered PCBs, in comparison to only 1 in 73 controls. In addition, 146 of 184 test animals developed preneoplastic lesions in their livers.

Although much work remains to define the carcinogenic effects of PCBs and to establish the likelihood of human susceptibility, it appears that PCBs are relatively weak carcinogens. While PCB contamination in the environment in the United States has been widespread and in some cases quite significant, liver cancer is relatively rare in the United States.

PCBs appear to play a relatively minor direct role in human carcinogenesis. However, the possible effects of these substances on the metabolism of other more potent environmental carcinogens should not be overlooked.

5. *Outbreak*

As is the case with many other environmental pollutants, documentation of the acute toxicity of PCBs in people has resulted from the widespread contamination of human food resulting from industrial accidents. In 1978 in Japan, the disease known as yusho occurred in Japan as a result of the contamination of rice oil with 2000–3000 ppm of PCB. The contamination resulted from a discharge of PCB heat transfer fluid into water that was subsequently used to irrigate rice fields. Over 1000 people showed symptoms of chloracne, pigmentation of the skin and nails, eye discharge, generalized swelling, weakness, vomiting, diarrhea, and weight loss. Growth rate retardation occurred in young children and in the fetuses of mothers who were exposed to the PCB. Again—as was the the case with rhesus monkeys—these effects were slow to dissipate, lasting in many cases from several months to a year following the initial exposure.

B. *Tetrachlorodibenzo-p-dioxin*

The chlorinated dibenzo-*p*-dioxins are among the most potent toxins known. The present concern about these compounds and the potential human health hazard they pose is a result of a growing awareness of their extraordinary toxicity and their inadvertent dispersion in the environment as trace contaminants of important commercial chemicals.

Dioxins are a large class of natural and synthetic substances that contain oxygen atoms held in ether linkages to carbon atoms generally within a six-membered ring. One comparatively small group of these substances, the dibenzodioxins, are of toxicological interest. The most notorious of the dioxins is tetrachlorodibenzo-*p*-dioxin (TCDD). Although TCDD has 22 different isomers that generally occur in mixtures in the environment, the 2,3,7,8-tetrachloro isomer (Figure 7.2) has received the greatest attention because of its unusual degree of toxicity.

At room temperature TCDD is a colorless crystalline solid; it melts at 305°C and is chemically quite stable, requiring temperatures of over 700°C before chemical decomposition occurs. It is lipophilic and binds strongly to solids and other particulate matter that occurs in soils. The compound is sparingly soluble in water and most organic liquids.

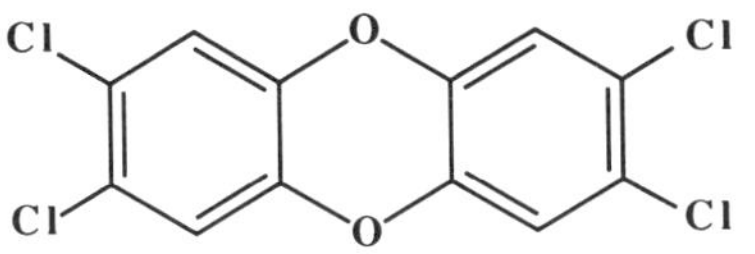

Figure 7.2 Structure of tetrachlorodibenzo-*p*-dioxin (TCDD).

1. Occurrence

The chlorinated dibenzo-*p*-dioxins are formed from the condensation of two orthochlorophenates. The particular dibenzo-*p*-dioxin formed depends on the chlorophenols present. In the commercial synthesis of the herbicide 2,4,5-trichlorophenate (2,4,5-T), the first step is the conversion of 1,2,4,5-tetrachlorobenzene to 2,4,5-trichlorophenate (Figure 7.3). At high temperatures an unwanted contaminant, 2,3,7,8-tetrachlorodibenzo-*p*-dioxin, is formed by the condensation of two trichloropenate molecules.

Herbicide synthesis is apparently not the only cause of environmental TCDD contamination. Significant levels of TCDD have been found in the incinerator smokestacks of chemical companies, even those that are not involved in the production of herbicides. Many reactions occur whenever organic and chlorine-containing substances are burned together. Some of these reactions apparently produce trace amounts of TCDD and various other dioxins.

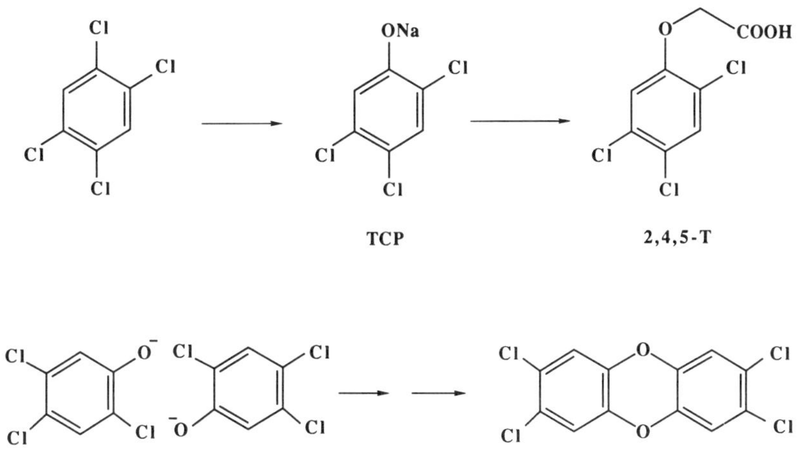

TCP

2,4,5-T

TCDD

Figure 7.3 Formation pathways of 2,4,5-T and TCDD.

2. *Mode of Toxic Action and Toxicities*

TCDD produces a wide range of physiological effects in humans and experimental animals. The guinea pig is the most sensitive species with an oral LD_{50} under 1 mg/kg. The hamster, the least sensitive species tested, has an LD_{50} some 10,000 times greater than that of the guinea pig. TCDD causes many effects in treated animals and the severity of these effects varies from species to species. For example, rats die from liver damage, but in the guinea pig the liver lesions seem less serious and the animals appear to succumb to a starvation-like wasting of the adrenals. The most common manifestation of TCDD poisoning is chloracne, which has been observed in rabbits, mice, monkeys, horses, and humans. Chloracne generally develops within 2–3 weeks following exposure and, depending on the severity of the exposure, may take from several months to many years to clear up. Kidney abnormalities appear in many species, and the extent of the lesions has prompted some researchers to conclude that the kidney is a specific target organ for TCDD exposure. Other physiological changes that have been observed in animal tests include hypothalamic atrophy, loss of fingernails and eyelashes, edema, bone marrow infection, polyneuropathy, and dry, scaly skin.

The carcinogenic effects of TCDD have been studied in some detail. TCDD enhances carcinogenic potency of several carcinogens when TCDD is administered following administration of the carcinogen. It is thus a promoter of carcinogenesis. It is also itself an extremely potent carcinogen. Results of an experiment with rats treated with 10 or 100 ng of TCDD/kg body weight showed greatly increased numbers of liver tumors. At the higher dose level, both male and female rats developed increased numbers of tumors of the mouth, nose, lungs, and liver. In female rats, TCDD is three times as potent a carcinogen as aflatoxin B_1, which is considered one of the most potent hepatocarcinogens known. The no effect level for TCDD in rats appears to be 10 ng/kg.

TCDD is a highly potent teratogen in mice and rabbits. Rabbits that received a range of doses below 1 mg/kg during the 6th to 15th day of pregnancy showed increased resorption, and higher rates of postimplantation loss. These effects were dose dependent. Severe effects on the bones and internal organs of surviving offspring were also apparent.

Results of small-scale studies with rhesus monkeys show that TCDD is fetotoxic to this species as well. Breeding monkeys fed TCDD at 1.7 ng/kg body weight per day for 2 years aborted four of seven pregnancies. Higher doses of TCDD produced higher levels of abortion and death in the pregnant females.

Although the results of experiments with laboratory animals clearly indicate the high toxicity, teratogenicity, and probable genotoxicity of TCDD, the outcomes of accidental human exposures suggest that people may be less sensitive to the toxic affects of TCDD than animal species. Many hundreds of cases of industrial accidents have been reported in which workers have been exposed to relatively high single doses of TCDD. In addition, approximately 37,000 residents of Seveso, Italy, may have been exposed to TCDD as a result of an accident in trichlorophenol manufacture that occurred in 1976. By far the most significant finding from the industrial exposures and from the Seveso incident is that humans are much less sensitive to the immediate toxic effects of TCDD than are guinea pigs. To date there has been no case of human fatality caused unequivocally by TCDD exposure. There are, however, many well-documented toxic effects in humans. Again, chloracne is the most obvious and initial effect in humans.

Other symptoms that develop with increased exposure include a general sense of fatigue, disturbances in the responses of the peripheral nervous system (such as a reduction in the speed at which nerve impulses travel through the limbs), and liver toxicity, including enlargement of the organ as well as changes in the levels of many enzymes. Data from industrial exposures indicate that these conditions generally disappear after a few years, and the experience at Seveso seems largely to confirm these findings in the general population.

Further evidence to suggest that humans are a good deal less sensitive to the toxic effects of TCDD than are animals comes from an incident that occurred in Missouri in 1982 where waste chemicals containing high levels of TCDD were combined with oils and used as dust retardants in horse arenas and stables. Although many rodents, including rats and mice, as well as larger animals, such as cats and dogs and many horses, died, apparently as a result of TCDD exposure, there were no incidences of human deaths. One child who used the soil of the arenas as a sandbox became ill, but the symptoms of the illness subsided with no obvious continued effects.

The most important question in regard to TCDD toxicity may be related to the long-term human effects of TCDD exposure and its possible teratogenic effects. Claims have been made about the teratogenic effects of the substance from Vietnam veterans who have been exposed to TCDD and from a group of people living in an area of Oregon where 2,4,5-T was routinely used to control undergrowth during forestry operations. However, teratogenic effects of TCDD in people have not been established. Results of a few well-controlled studies have suggested a role of TCDD exposure in formation of cancers of soft tissue in humans. The work of a Swedish group linked the use of TCDD-contaminated phenoxy herbicides with increased sarcomas of muscles, nerves, and fat tissue in people. In two studies, five- to sixfold increases in the incidences of this type of tumor were observed in people exposed to phenoxy herbicides compared to an unexposed control group. Although the validity of these studies has been criticized on several grounds, other studies of mortality rates in chemical workers exposed to TCDD through industrial accidents also show an increased level of soft tissue sarcoma.

In summary, then, TCDD has been shown to be one of the most toxic and carcinogenic substances in various animal species, and it occurs at low levels in apparently widespread areas of the environment. Humans appear to be quite resistant to the acute affects of TCDD. Much of this apparent resistance may be because humans ingest very small levels of TCDD in comparison to the levels that are administered to experimental animals. Several analyses of fish, milk, water, and beef fat used for human consumption were unable to detect TCDD at a detection limit of 1 ppt. Human exposures have been mainly through the skin. Evidence implicating TCDD exposure in the occurrence of soft tissue sarcomas in people is cause for concern and justifies efforts to minimize human exposure to this substance.

II. Heavy Metals

A. Lead

1. *Occurrence*

Lead, occurring chiefly as the sulfide, galena, is the most abundant of the heavy metals found in the earth's crust. The heating process required to convert the ore to metal was used by the early Phoenicians, Egyptians, Greeks, Chinese, and East Indians in the preparation of eating utensils, water ducts, vessels for various liquids, ornaments, and weights. The early Romans used lead for their extensive aqueduct system and for storage vessels for wine and food. Some historians have suggested that the extensive use of lead-containing vessels by the Romans may have contributed to mental and emotional instability in Roman leaders and thus to the downfall of the Roman Empire. Reports by ancient Roman physicians show that roughly two-thirds of the emperors who reigned between 30 B.C. and 220 A.D. drank a great deal of lead-tainted wine and that most of them had gout, a condition occasionally reported in lead poisoning due to moonshine whiskey and indicative of lead-induced kidney deterioration. The most likely source of lead was the addition to Roman wines of boiled-down grape syrup prepared in lead-lined vessels. Contemporary efforts to prepare the syrup according to the ancient recipes yielded a mixture with 240–1000 mg of lead/liter. Thus, very high levels of lead could occur in the wine from the combined practices of using lead-lined vessels for wine storage and consumption, and by the use of lead-tainted syrup in wine preparation.

2. *Environmental Contamination*

The principal causes of environmental lead contamination in recent times stem from its use in lead storage batteries and as gasoline anti-knock additives. Lead-containing pesticides have also been used, but this use has decreased in recent years.

In the early 1970s, typical premium gasoline contained between 2 and 4 g of lead per gallon with an average of about 2.8 g. Regular gasoline averaged about 2.3 g of lead per gallon. Thus, in California, where over 13 million motor vehicles were in use, the total lead consumed in gasoline was approximately 26,000 tons per year. On the average 70 to 80% of the lead in gasoline is exhausted out the tailpipe as particulate. Less is exhausted at low-speed driving and more is exhausted under freeway conditions.

During the early 1970s there was intense public debate over the question of whether or not lead should be banned from gasoline. The issue was resolved when the automobile industry met lower the automobile emissions standards, resulting in a reduction of airborne lead in busy traffic cities such as New York.

Lead occurs widely throughout the environment and has been found in all bodies of water and soils tested. The major non-industrial sources of lead contamination for people are food and water. Supplies of drinking water for most cities in the Unites States contain levels of lead considerably lower than the 50 μg/liter maximum allowed by the U.S. Public Health Service. However, water that has been allowed to stand in lead pipes or in lead-containing vessels for periods of only a few days may contain lead in concentrations of 1 mg/liter.

3. *Food Contamination*

Lead has been detected in all foods examined, even those grown far from industrialized areas. Recent analyses suggest a natural level of lead to be on the order of 0.3 ppb in wide-ranging marine fish. These fish are comparatively free of geographically localized contamination and are considered good indicators of general environmental contamination. Levels considerably in excess of this, however, have been detected in commonly consumed foods. In general, plant foods grown in industrialized areas and near freeways contain significantly higher levels of lead than foods grown in remote areas. For example, bean pods and corn husks grown in a rural area of Mexico had lead levels of 0.04 and 0.26 ppm, respectively, while these same plant components obtained from urban gardens near highways had lead levels at least 10 times higher. For animal products, the highest levels of lead are found in bone; as a food group, seafood tends to contain the highest levels of lead, with a range of 0.2–2.5 ppm. On the average, the total lead intake from food is estimated to be in the range of 0.2–0.4 mg/day, whereas from water the estimate is roughly 0.01 mg/day.

In the past, lead-soldered cans were a well-known source of lead, contaminating such food products as infant formulas, evaporated milk, infant juices, and baby foods. Lead levels of 0.5 ppm in these products were not uncommon. Analyses of albacore indicate that conventional processing of food increases considerably the lead levels in the canned product. Butchering and packing the albacore in unsoldered cans results in a 20-fold increase in the levels of lead, while butchering, grinding, air drying, and packing result in a 400-fold increase. A 4000-fold increase in lead levels of albacore results from butchering and packing in lead-soldered cans. In the United States, the FDA and the canning industry have combined efforts to institute the use of non-soldered cans. The result has been a drop in lead levels in products used primarily by infants to one-fifth to one-tenth the levels observed when soldered cans were used.

4. Mode of Toxic Action

The extent of lead absorption in the gastrointestinal tract depends on several factors. One factor is the chemical form of the lead. Organic lead compounds, such as tetraethyllead, are readily absorbed from the gastrointestinal tract (> 90%), eventually concentrating primarily in the bone, and to a lesser extent in the liver, kidney, muscle, and central nervous system. Under normal circumstances in the adult, inorganic lead compounds are poorly absorbed from the alimentary tract (5–10%). Absorption of inorganic lead in infants and children is considerably higher, however, with estimates in the range of 40–50%. Absorbed lead is excreted primarily in the urine (75%) and feces (16%).

Several dietary factors affect the level of lead absorption in people and experimental animals. For example, approximately three times as much lead is absorbed following a 16-hr fast than when lead is administered following a normal period of food or feed consumption. In animal studies, increasing the corn oil content of the diet from 5 to 40% results in a 7- to 14-fold increase in lead content in many tissues. Low levels of dietary calcium produce increased levels of lead absorption and resultant lead toxicity. Lead exposure of rats consuming diets low but not deficient in calcium produced 4-fold higher blood lead levels than in lead-exposed rats consuming a diet with adequate calcium levels. This is because calcium appears to compete with lead in the gastrointestinal tract for a common absorption site. Iron deficiency also affects lead absorption from the gastrointestinal tract. As much as 6-fold increases in tissue lead have been reported for rats in which iron stores had been reduced. Decreased zinc intakes also result in increased gastrointestinal absorption of lead and increased toxicity of lead. Zinc is also reported to influence lead levels in the fetuses of animals that have been treated with lead.

Dietary factors and aging may also affect distribution of lead in the body. A low-calcium diet limits the amount of lead that can be stored in bone because bone formation is slower. Under normal circumstances lead has a biological half-life of about 10,000 days in bone. At times of low calcium intake, however, a significant amount of lead may be released from the bone because of bone resorption. The stored lead is then released into the blood stream. Under such conditions higher lead content in the kidney and blood has been observed in experiments with animals. This may prove especially significant for elderly people. Aging is frequently accompanied by bone demineralization and previously immobilized lead may be released. The higher incidence of kidney disease and urinary problems in the elderly further increases susceptibility to lead poisoning since urinary excretion of lead is inhibited.

Three stages of lead poisoning have been recognized. The first stage, called the asymptomatic stage, is generally not associated with behavioral disorders or organ dysfunction, but is characterized by changes in the blood. Anemia is a well-established early symptom of relatively mild lead poisoning. Lead decreases the lifetime of erythrocytes and the synthesis of heme. Although the interaction of lead with the hematopoietic system is quite complex (Figure 7.4), most of the observed effects of lead on blood can be explained by its inhibitory influences on δ-aminolevulinic acid (ALA) synthetase, ALA dehydrase, and ferrochelatase. Stage 1 of lead poisoning is characterized by an increase of uroporphyrinogen III level in the blood resulting from decreased insertion of iron into uroporphyrinogen III mediated by ferrochelatase. Also at this stage, urinary ALA is increased since the ALA dehydrase-mediated conversion of ALA to prophobilinogen is decreased. In the later phases of this asymptomatic

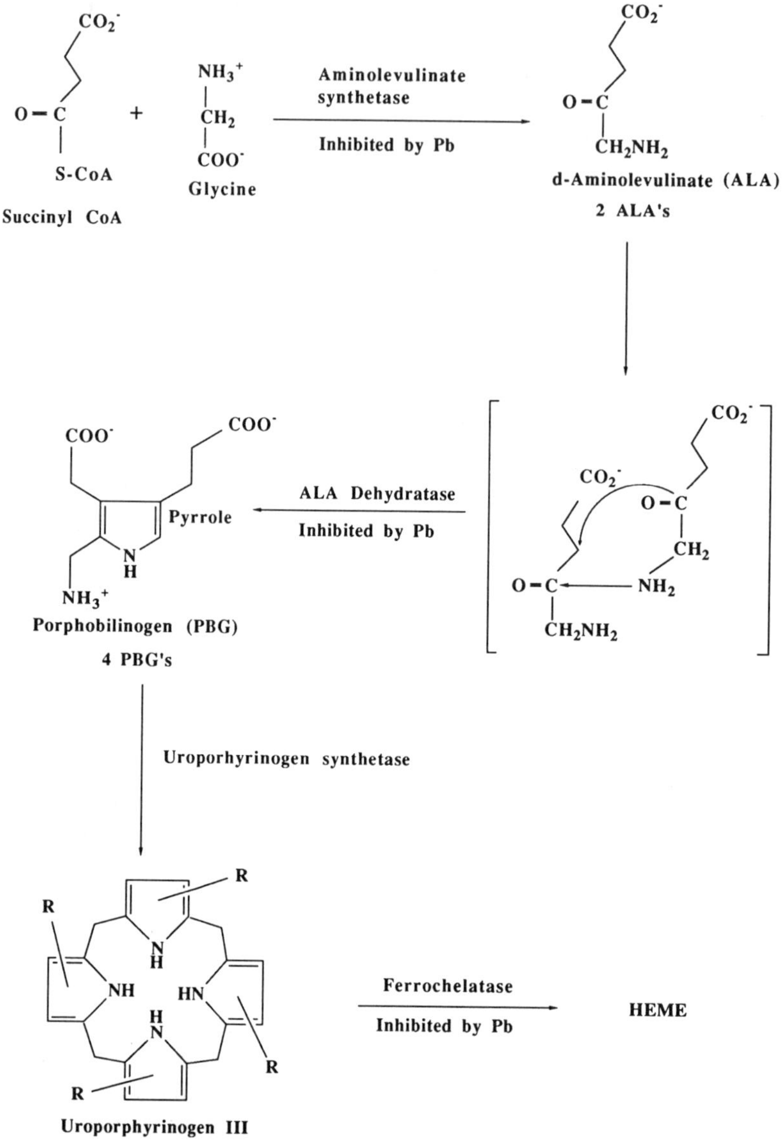

CO_2^-

O−C + NH_3^+ — CH_2 — COO^-

S-CoA

Glycine

Succinyl CoA

Aminolevulinate synthetase

Inhibited by Pb

CO_2^-

O−C

CH_2NH_2

d-Aminolevulinate (ALA)

2 ALA's

COO⁻ COO⁻

Pyrrole

N H

NH_3^+

Porphobilinogen (PBG)

4 PBG's

ALA Dehydratase

Inhibited by Pb

CO_2^-

CO_2^-

O−C

CH_2

O−C — NH_2

CH_2NH_2

Uroporhyrinogen synthetase

R R

NH HN

N H

H N

R R

Uroporphyrinogen III

Ferrochelatase

Inhibited by Pb

HEME

Figure 7.4 Mechanisms of heme synthesis.

period, urinary ALA is further increased and hematocrit and hemoglobin values decrease.

In Stage II lead poisoning, the symptomatic stage or the symptomatic period, anemia may be quite obvious, and disorders of the central nervous system, including hyperactivity, impulsive behavior, perceptual disorders, and slowed learning ability, appear. In more severe cases, the symptoms include restlessness, irritability, headaches, muscular tremor, ataxia, and loss of memory. With continued exposure to lead, Stage III ensues with symptoms that may culminate in kidney failure, convulsions, coma, and death. These symptoms have been reported in industrial accidents or following consumption of house paint or moonshine whiskey.

Of major concern are the neurological effects produced in children by continued exposure to relatively low levels of lead. In one study designed to assess the magnitude of this problem, groups of school children were placed into low-lead and high-lead exposure groups according to the lead level found in deciduous teeth. Although none of the children exhibited the symptoms of clinical lead poisoning, children in the high-lead group showed increased distractibility, inability to follow directions, and increased impulsivity compared to children in the low-lead group. Children in the high-lead group also scored lower on standard IQ tests and verbal tests.

The levels of lead in the blood associated with various symptoms are indicated in Table 7.1. A dose within the range of 0.2–2.0 mg lead/day in the adult human is generally required to produce measurable effects in the blood and to produce blood lead levels in the range of 20–30 mg/dl. However, in a child 1–3 years of age, consumption of approximately 135 mg/day with 50% absorption from the gastrointestinal tract results

TABLE 7.1
Symptoms of Lead in Blood

Level of Pb in blood (mg/100 ml)	Symptoms
25–30	Protoporphyrin increase in blood, ALA increase in urine
40–50	Hematocrit decrease, hemoglobin decrease, ALA increase
50–60	Anemia
>60	Hyperkinesis, short attention span, aggressive conduct (minimal brain disfunction)
>120	Mental retardation, blindness, death

in approximately 20 μg/dl in the blood. The actual levels of lead consumption from the diet, estimated to be in the order of 0.2–0.4 mg/day for adults and 0.1 mg/day for infants, are in the range of doses that produce measurable effects in blood and may be in excess of the doses required to adversely affect neurological functions.

These dangerously high levels of lead consumption, especially for children, have been pointed out by many scientists, and the problem has been clearly described by a panel of the National Academy of Sciences. The consensus of scientific opinion is that human exposure to lead must be reduced wherever possible.

B. Mercury

1. Occurrence

Mercury occurs primarily in geographical belts in the earth's crust as its red sulfide, cinnabar. The heating process required to prepare free metallic mercury from its sulfide was discovered in very early times. Because of its shiny, fluid appearance and its very great density, magical powers were attributed to metallic mercury; as a result, mercury was put to many questionable uses in alchemy and medicine. Although metallic mercury was used until relatively recent times to remedy bowel obstructions, it is no longer used in remedies in modern medicine.

For economic reasons and because of the now well-established toxicity of mercury and many of its derivatives, uses of mercury today are quite restricted, and there is an increased effort to reprocess and reclaim mercury used in many products. Metallic mercury and mercury salts are used primarily by the electrical and chemical industries in switches, coatings, and catalysts. Organomercurial compounds are used to some extent as diuretics, but are being increasingly replaced by nonmercurial compounds. Also, organomercurials in various forms are very popular antiseptics and are used in some cases in sterilizing solutions for medical instruments. Mercury continues to be used in the dental preparations for fillings. Projections for world mercury use by the year 2000 are in the range of 10^5 kg/year.

Until relatively recent times mercury was thought to be environmentally stable, so discarded metallic mercury was simply buried in the ground or deposited in waterways. In addition, salts of mercury were thought to readily form complexes with various components in water and to form inert precipitates. However, as indicated in Figure 7.5, mercury can be converted from one form to another in the environment.

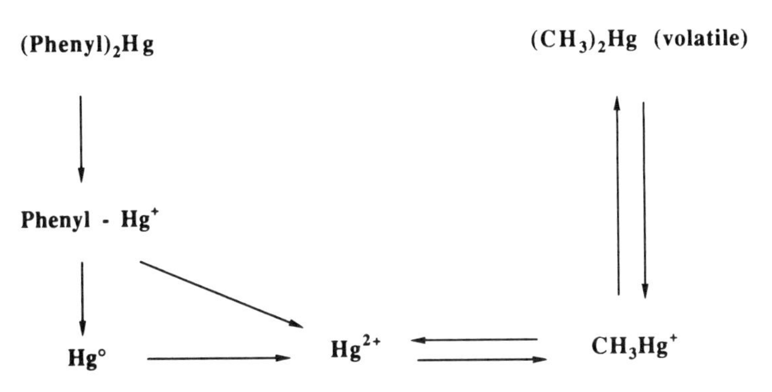

Figure 7.5 Mercury conversion pathways.

Metallic mercury deposited in a lake settles into the sediment where bacteria may carry out oxidations and alkylations producing both water-soluble substances (salts) and lipid-soluble substances (alk·' compounds). The dialkyl mercury compounds are relatively volatile and can be transported in the air. These metabolic conversions, therefore, provide a means whereby mercury deposited in one form in the environment will eventually be converted to another form and may be found at sites distant from the original site of disposal. For example, a highly toxic organomercurial compound used primarily as an algacide will eventually be converted, at least in part, to the less toxic inorganic forms and to metallic mercury. In addition, such organomercurial compounds are eventually converted to methyl mercury, the most toxic of the mercurial compounds.

2. Contamination in Foods

Mercury contamination of food depends to a great extent on the chemical form that is placed in the environment or the extent of environmental interconversion of mercury compounds. Mercury levels of most plant foods and meats are generally considered to be quite low, with recent estimates for meats produced in the United States indicating a range of 1–7 ppb. Mercury levels of other food including potatoes, legumes, and cereals are generally less than 50 ppb. In the few cases that have been examined, methyl mercury accounts for the greatest percentage of mercury compounds in meat products, and in fish. Inorganic mercury is thought to be the major form of mercury in plant foods.

Fish is the primary source of dietary mercury. Fish and other creatures, such as predatory birds, which occupy advanced levels in the food chain, are known to concentrate mercury as much as 1000-fold above the levels that occur in their immediate environment. Larger marine fish have higher concentrations of mercury than smaller fish. For example, analyses by the FDA indicate that large tuna contain an average of 0.25 ppm of mercury while smaller tuna have an average of 0.13 ppm. In addition, the amount of methyl mercury relative to total mercury increases with the age of the fish. Shellfish accumulate mercury from the aquatic environment at levels nearly 3000 times greater than the levels to which they are exposed in the water. Analyses of fish in many countries indicate that 99% of the world's fish catch has a total mercury content not exceeding 0.5 mg/kg.

The FDA has set this level of 0.5 ppm as a maximum acceptable level of mercury in fish and shellfish, and the World Health Organization (WHO) recommended a maximum level of mercury of 0.05 ppm mercury in food items other than fish. Based on analyses of mercury levels associated with human poisoning, a committee of the WHO has suggested a provisional tolerable intake of mercury of 0.3 mg total/week that is not to include more than 0.2 mg of methyl mercury. Thus, weekly consumption of about 600 g (or approximately 86 g/day) of fish containing 0.5 mg/kg of mercury would not exceed the tolerable intake. According to a 1972 report by the WHO, per capita fish consumption in Sweden was 56 g/day, 18 g/day in the United States, and 88 g/day in Japan. These data indicate that potentially large numbers of individuals are consuming enough fish to put them at risk of mercury poisoning.

Because of the dramatic and tragic demonstrations of the acute effects of mercury poisoning in humans, regulatory agencies throughout the world became concerned about the natural levels of mercury in the diet. Extensive analyses of fish in the United States and elsewhere revealed that mercury levels far in excess of the 0.5 ppm guidelines occur in commonly consumed species. For example, in Lake Erie, levels as high as 10 ppm were found in some fish. Larger marine fish also were consistently found to have mercury levels in excess of the 0.5 ppm. Swordfish in particular were incriminated when analyses revealed that only a small percentage of the total samples of this fish had levels of mercury less than 0.5 ppm. As a result, in 1971 the FDA seized over 800,000 pounds of commercial swordfish, which led to the near collapse of the swordfish industry in the United States and elsewhere. These apparently high levels of mercury in marine fish were blamed on contemporary pollution of the marine environment until analyses of museum specimens of fish revealed that the levels of mercury had not changed significantly over the past 100 years. In addition, mercury in fish is less toxic than mercury by itself. The toxicity is reduced by selenium that occurs along with the mercury in fish at an approximate 1:1 ratio. These as yet unexplained phenomena are the subjects of continuing research.

3. In Vivo *Absorption and Toxicity*

The extent of absorption of mercury compounds is dependent on the site of absorption and the chemical form of the element. Less than 0.01% of ingested metallic mercury is absorbed from the gastrointestinal tract. Thus, the use of metallic mercury in the treatment of bowel obstruction was probably of little hazard. However, approximately 80% of inhaled metallic mercury in the vapor state is absorbed in the respiratory tract. Estimates of absorption of mercury salts range from approximately 2% of the daily intake of mercuric chloride in mice to approximately 20% of mercuric acetate in rats.

Absorption and distribution of alkyl mercury compounds, because of their greater lipid solubility, are much more extensive than for either of the inorganic forms. Results of experiments with human volunteers and with several animal species indicate that methyl mercury is absorbed almost completely from the gastrointestinal tract. Following absorption, methyl mercury moves to the plasma, where it is bound in the red blood cells. The compound then moves primarily to the kidneys, as well as to the colon, muscles, and other tissues, including those of the fetus. Concentrations of methyl mercury in fetal blood are increased over concentrations in maternal blood. This apparently is due to the increased concentration of hemaglobin in the fetal blood. Although total transport across the blood–brain barrier is relatively slow, removal of methyl mercury from the brain appears to lag behind removal from other tissues; the concentration of methyl mercury in the brain is roughly 10 times higher than that in the blood for people.

Most mercury compounds are metabolized to the mercuric state and excreted in the urine and feces. In contrast, methyl mercury is excreted mainly in the feces by processes of biliary excretion and exfoliation of intestinal epithelial cells. Extensive reabsorption of methyl mercury from the intestines is one of the factors increasing the biological half-life (80 days) of this compound.

Toxic effects of mercury compounds in humans have been known for many years. Inorganic mercury affects primarily the kidney, effected by inorganic mercury leading to uremia and anuria. The early symptoms of acute inorganic mercury poisoning are gastrointestinal upset, abdominal pain, nausea, vomiting, and bloody diarrhea. Doses required for acute kidney effects appear to be in excess of 175 ppm of mercuric salts in the diet.

4. Outbreaks

Perhaps the first well-established incidences of poisoning from organomercurial compounds involving relatively large numbers of people began in 1954 in Japan. Severe neuromuscular and neurological defects began to appear in people living near Minamata Bay and later in people living near Niigata, Japan. In these two locations as of 1970, poisoning of over 120 people was officially documented with 50 deaths reported. Early symptoms of methyl mercury poisoning, also dubbed Minamata disease, include loss of sensation at the extremities of the fingers and toes and areas around the mouth, loss of coordination, slurred speech, a diminution of vision called tunnel vision, and loss of hearing. Pregnant women exposed to methyl mercury gave birth to infants with mental retardation and cerebral palsy. Later symptoms include progressive blindness, deafness, lack of coordination, and mental deterioration. Neuromuscular development is abnormal in individuals exposed *in utero*. The cause of the disease was traced to consumption of fish from the local waters that were heavily contaminated with methyl mercury. Chemical factories that were located upstream from these towns were the source of the methyl mercury that eventually accumulated in the fish.

During the decades of the 1950s, 1960s, and 1970s, several outbreaks of human poisoning due to consumption of wheat products treated with mercury pesticides were reported with many thousands of individuals affected. In an incident of methyl mercury poisoning that occurred in 1972 in Iraq, 6530 people were officially admitted to hospitals and 459 of these patients died. The outbreak occurred as a result of consumption of bread made from seed wheat. The seed, treated with methyl mercury fungicide and colored with a brownish-red dye, was distributed in bags that were labeled in English and marked with appropriate warnings. Farmers were apparently not familiar with the warnings, and the brownish-red dye could be removed by washing, giving the impression that the poison was removed. The seed was ground into flour and subsequently used to make bread.

C. Cadmium

1. Occurrence

Cadmium has chemical characteristics similar to those of zinc. Cadmium occurs in nature wherever zinc is found and is produced as a by-product in the mining of zinc and lead. It is used in the galvanizing of other metals to prevent rusting and in the manufacture of storage batteries and plastics.

The major sources of cadmium exposure for the general population are water, food, and tobacco. The ultimate source of contamination of these products is difficult to discover. Cadmium in water often results from the cadmium alloys used to galvanize water pipes. However, no single source of cadmium contamination in the environment has been identified.

Food generally contains less than 0.05 ppm of cadmium, providing an estimated 0.5 mg cadmium/week. Analyses of the world food supply conducted on a periodic basis by the World Health Organization indicate that the foods with the highest levels of cadmium contamination are consistently shellfish and kidneys of various animals including cattle, chicken, pigs, sheep, and turkeys. Cadmium levels in kidneys, for example, are often in excess of 10 ppm, while cadmium levels in shellfish, such as oysters, reach levels as high as 200–300 ppm. Cadmium levels are about 0.03 ppm in most meats in the Untied States and 0.075 ppm in hamburger. The higher levels of cadmium in the hamburger are probably due to processing methods. Soybeans are reported to contain 0.09 ppm cadmium while most other plant foods are very low in cadmium (e.g., 0.003 ppm in apples).

When considered as part of the normal diet, these various dietary components provide an estimated 73 μg cadmium/day per person. This value is not significantly different from the provisional tolerable intake set by the WHO (57–71 μg/day). The provisional allowable intake has been developed based on the results of experiments with animals and on analyses of human exposures in industrial accidents resulting in cadmium poisoning. The value includes a safety margin of a factor of approximately four from a level that can cause minimal kidney damage with long-term consumption. Thus, the levels of cadmium present in the diet do not appear to present an imminent health hazard to people in a general population. However, for individuals who consume unusually large amounts of shellfish or kidneys, the daily intake of cadmium may be in excess of provisional tolerable intake.

2. In Vivo *Absorption and Toxicity*

Data on the biological effects of cadmium in people are incomplete compared to data for mercury and lead. Apparently only about 5% of orally administered cadmium is absorbed in the gastrointestinal tract. The various salts of cadmium differ in their water solubility, and, therefore, may be absorbed to somewhat differing extents. Cadmium does not occur as stable alkyl derivatives that would be expected to have increased lipid solubility. The extent of absorption of cadmium from the gastrointestinal tract of rats is considerably greater in the newborn animal than in the older animal. Rats dosed with cadmium fluoride at 2 and 24 hr of age absorbed over 20 and 10 times, respectively, the amount of cadmium absorbed by animals dosed at 6 weeks of age. In addition, the extent of absorption was dependent on other factors. For example, the absorption of cadmium taken with milk was roughly 20 times greater than absorption of cadmium taken without milk. For humans the extent of cadmium absorption can double under the influence of calcium, protein, or zinc deficiency.

Distribution of cadmium has been studied in laboratory animals. In rats, absorbed cadmium is distributed to the liver, spleen, adrenals, and duodenum within 48 hr following administration. Accumulation is slower in the kidneys, where peak levels are reached by the sixth day. Unless the dose of cadmium is unusually high, levels in the kidneys are roughly 10 times the levels in the liver. With very high doses, the levels of cadmium in these two organs become similar. With continued low doses, concentrations of cadmium in the other organs remain small, with about 50% of the total cadmium in the body occurring in the kidneys and liver.

Cadmium is highly stable in the body with estimates of biological half-life ranging from 20 to 40 years. It is thought that a metal-binding protein, known as metallothionein, present in the kidneys is responsible for cadmium's long biological half-life. Metallothionein synthesis is increased in response to cadmium and zinc exposure. As the levels of cadmium increase in the body, so do the levels of metallothionein. It is not clear, however, why the kidneys are the major site of cadmium concentration since metallothionein is present in several other organs as well. Also, metallothionein in itself does not reduce the toxicity of cadmium. The cadmium–metallothionein complex is actually more toxic than cadmium alone.

Biological effects of cadmium have been studied extensively in rats. In these studies the most sensitive organ to cadmium exposure is the kidney, with symptoms of toxicity arising in rats at a dose of 0.25 mg/kg. Symptoms include increased excretion of glucose, protein, amino acids, calcium, and uric acid. The liver is also affected as indicated by increased gluconeogenesis, leading to hyperglycemia, and pancreatic effects are indicated by a decreased circulating insulin level. At higher doses (2 mg/kg), the testes and prostate glands atrophy and the adrenals hypertrophy with increased levels of circulating epinephrine and norepinephrine. Also, there is evidence of increased levels of dopamine in the brain. There are some indications that cadmium is a hypertensive agent, a teratogen, and a carcinogen, although these results have not been confirmed in humans.

Several components in the diet reduce or eliminate some of the toxic effects of cadmium. Zinc, selenium, copper, iron, and ascorbic acid are protective agents. The mechanism by which these protective effects occur is by no means clear.

3. Outbreaks

Cadmium has been implicated as the cause of at least one epidemic of human disease resulting from contaminated food. This epidemic occurred in the Jintsu River Valley of Japan following World War II. Local health practitioners observed many cases of kidney damage and skeletal disorders accompanied by great pain. The disease was called in Japanese itai-itai byo, which is loosely translated as ouch-ouch disease. It was soon realized that certain other host factors in addition to consumption of contaminated food were required to initiate the disease. These other host factors include pregnancy, lactation, aging, and calcium deficiency. The dietary source of human cadmium poisoning was thought to be contaminated rice that had cadmium levels of 120–350 ppm of ash, compared to 20 ppm of rice ash in the control area. The source of this cadmium was thought to be a lead–zinc–cadmium mine upstream from the rice fields. Although the weight of scientific opinion is consistent with the idea that cadmium is involved in the etiology of itai-itai disease, reservations about this hypothesis have been raised by several investigators. One piece of evidence that certainly suggests that cadmium is not the only causative agent of the disease is that high levels of cadmium are found in rice from many areas of Japan where no cases of the disease have been reported.

Suggestions for Further Reading

1. Bornschein, R., Pearson, D., and Reiter, L. (1980). Behavioral effects of moderate lead exposure in children and animals models. I. Clinical studies. *CRC Crit Rev. Toxicol.*, **43.**
2. D'Itri, F. M., and Kamrin, M. A. (eds.) (1983). "PCBs, Human and Environmental Hazards." Butterworth Publishers, Boston.
3. Graham, H. (ed.) (1980). "The Safety of Foods," 2nd Ed. AVI Publishing Company. Westport, Connecticut.
4. Kehoe, R. (1976). Pharmacology and toxicology of heavy metals; lead. *Pharmacol. Ther.* **1,** 161.
5. Kopps, S., Gloned, T., Perry, H., Jr., Erlanger, M., and Perry, E. (1982). Cardiovascular actions of cadmium at environmental exposure levels. *Science* **217,** 837.
6. Mahaffery, K. R., (1981). Nutritional factors in lead poisoning. *Nutr. Rev.* **39,** 353.
7. Poland, A., and Knutson, J. (1982). 2,3,7,8-Tetrachlorodibenzo-p-dioxin and related halogenated aromatic hydrocarbons: examination of the mechanism of toxicity. *Annu. Rev. Pharmacol. Toxicol.* **22,** 517.

8. Rice, D., and Gilbert, S. (1982). Early chronic low-level methyl mercury poisoning in monkeys impairs spatial vision. *Science* **216,** 759.
9. Robinson, J., and Tuovinen, O. (1984). Mechanisms of microbial resistance and detoxification of mercury and organomercury compounds: physiological, biochemical, and genetic analyses. *Microbiol. Rev.* **48,** 95.
10. Sielken, R., Jr. (1987). Quantitative cancer risk assessments for 2,3,7,8-tetrachlorodibenzo-p-dioxin (TCDD). *Food Chem. Toxicol.* **25:**257.
11. Singhal, R., Anderson, M., and Meister, A. (1987). Glutathione, a first line of defense against cadmium toxicity. *FASEB J.* **1,** 220.

CHAPTER **8**

Pesticide Residues in Foods

I. History

Pesticides, either synthetic or naturally occurring, are a diverse group of chemicals used to control undesirable effects of target organisms. Pesticides may be classified according to their target organisms. For food toxicology the important categories of target organisms are insecticides, fungicides, and herbicides. Acaricides (which affect mites), molluscicides, and rodenticides are less important.

Commercial production is a relatively recent innovation in the development of synthetic pesticides. As an example of this, the value of the insecticidal effects of DDT, which was synthesized in 1874, was not reported until 1939, after commercial production had begun. The Swiss chemist, Mueller, received a Nobel prize in 1948 for his discovery of the insecticidal effects of DDT. Its value to public health in controlling insect vectors of disease was demonstrated following World War II. In response to a shortage of nicotine during World War II in Germany, the first organophosphate insecticide, tetraethyl pyrophosphate (TEPP), was developed. Parathion, synthesized by the German scientist Schrader in 1944, was among the first insecticides of commercial importance and it continues to be widely used.

The introduction of these and other synthetic pesticides has made an enormous contribution not only to agriculture but also to human health. For example, in Europe and Asia during and after World War II, thousands of lives were saved by the use of DDT to control the mosquito vector of malaria transmission. The "green revolution" of recent decades (a dramatic increase in agricultural output) is a result of the use of synthetic pesticides to control weeds and insects that would otherwise limit crop production. Insecticides and fungicides are also used to reduce postharvest losses of valuable crops and to maintain the nutritional value and freshness of food until it is consumed. On the other hand, much attention has been turned to the possible hazards of pesticide residues in foods, which have become one of today's most important food safety issues.

Until quite recently, far too little attention was paid to toxic effects of pesticides on humans and other non-target organisms. This lack of concern has resulted in disastrous ecological consequences. For example, contamination of both groundwater and soil is now a serious problem in many agricultural areas of the United States. In some cases, contamination persists for decades after use of the offending product is discontinued. In the past, poor management practices were the cause of an extreme overuse of such pesticides as DDT, which in turn led to the development of resistance in target organisms.

Since the 1962 publication of Rachel Carson's book, *Silent Spring*, the role of pesticides in modern society has become an emotional and contentious issue. More recently, the controversy has broadened to include questions about the safety of pesticide residues in foods, which can now be analyzed in great detail as a result of dramatic increases in chemists' analytical capabilities.

II. Pesticides in the Food Chain

In recent years, contamination of surface and groundwater by pesticides has been recognized as a serious and growing problem in agricultural regions. While many pesticides degrade rapidly in the environment, bind tightly to soil, or are simply too insoluble or non-volatile to move throughout the environment, others are both persistent and mobile. Certain pesticide application methods, particularly aerial spraying, are notoriously inefficient in delivering the pesticide to the target. Large amounts enter the environment directly, and runoff from agricultural fields may contaminate both surface and groundwater. Livestock that drink the contaminated water may have detectable pesticide residues in their meat or milk.

In some areas, non-agricultural applications of pesticides may also be a source of environmental and water contamination. Home use of pesticides, which constitutes a significant percentage of total use of pesticides, is subject to the same laws and regulations as agricultural uses. However, although home use involves the least hazardous pesticides, the possibility of misuse by homeowners is significant. Not only can contamination of home-grown produce occur, but accidental poisoning due to improper storage and disposal happen often. Another example of non-agricultural application of pesticides is forest management, which often involves large quantities of herbicides and insecticides. Maintenance of golf courses and other expanses of turf is pesticide-intensive and often involves fungicides that pose a significant risk to mammals. Also, in many areas, commercial and recreational fishing is restricted because of environmental contamination by persistent pesticides.

To the extent that contaminated water is used in the processing or preparation of food, pesticides may enter the food supply through this medium. Human exposure to contaminated water through drinking or washing also has an indirect effect on issues of pesticide residues in foods since it may comprise a significant portion of pesticide contamination within the exposed population. Thousands of samples of food are examined by the FDA each year to determine compliance with established pesticide tolerances on raw agricultural products. Residues of pesticide chemicals are found in about half of the samples, and generally about 3% of the samples contain residues in excess of, or not authorized by, legal tolerances. Table 8.1 shows the residual amounts of some commonly used pesticides in food commodities.

III. Regulations

In the United States, the regulation of pesticides is under the jurisdiction of the Environmental Protection Agency (EPA), the Food and Drug Administration (FDA), and the United States Department of Agriculture

TABLE 8.1
Concentration (ppm) Range of Commonly Used Pesticides Found in Various Food Groups

Pesticides	Dairy products	Meat, fish, poultry	Grain, cereal
Captan	0	0	0
DDT	0	0.004–0.009	0
Dieldrin	trace–0.02	trace–0.002	0
Malathion	0	0	0.007–0.149
Methoxychlor	0.006	0	0
Parathion	0	0	0

(USDA). The EPA handles pesticide registration and the establishment of tolerances while the FDA and the USDA monitor pesticide residue levels in the food supply. Additionally, a number of states, most notably California and Texas, have implemented extensive regulation.

Under Section 408 of the Food, Drug and Cosmetics Act (FDCA), residues of pesticides on processed foods are regulated as food additives. Congress has specifically exempted residues on raw agricultural products from the scope of the FDCA. By law, no pesticide that will leave a detectable residue—whether of parent compound, breakdown product, or metabolite—in a processed food can be registered until a tolerance for such residue levels has been set by the EPA. For new products or uses, tolerances are set based on results of extensive toxicological testing. In general, a tolerance is set no higher than the "no observable effect level" (NOEL) found in such testing, divided by a safety factor of 100. However, if good agricultural practice can result in an even lower level of residues, the legal tolerance will be reduced accordingly.

Compounds that are considered possible or probable human carcinogens as a result of animal testing are regulated more stringently. Under Section 409 of the FDCA, specifically the Delaney Clause, no tolerance can be set for any carcinogen in processed foods. Without a tolerance, the compound then becomes an illegal food additive. The EPA's current practice is to deny a tolerance even for raw agricultural products since the Delaney Clause prohibits setting a Section 409 tolerance. Currently, these regulations do not apply to the pesticides that were in use before these laws were adopted. The EPA has required re-registration of such products, along with any additional toxicological testing required to meet current standards. Many compounds or uses will be eliminated when this program of re-registration is completed. However, in the meantime, these products remain in use, giving rise to much controversy.

The Department of Agriculture controls approval of pesticides for production under the Federal Insecticide, Fungicide, and Rodenticide Act (FIFRA) of 1964. This law provides that any "economic poison" or chemical pesticide must be registered before being marketed in interstate commerce.

The majority of components in most formulated pesticides are listed on the label only as "inert ingredients." These components include solvents, surfactants, carriers, antioxidants and other compounds; they are inert only insofar as they themselves exert no pesticidal action. Current pesticide regulation does not deal directly with "inert ingredients" nor their residues or possible toxic effects. Future amendments to FIFRA are likely to deal with this aspect of pesticide manufacture and use.

IV. Insecticides

A. DDT

Although DDT [1,1′–(2,2,2-trichloroethylidene)bis(4-chlorobenzene)] (Figure 8.1) has been banned in the United States since 1972, it remains one of the best-known synthetic pesticides. The incidence of malaria before and after the use of DDT is shown in Table 8.2. Because DDT is a very nonpolar molecule, it has high lipid solubility. Since DDT is also extremely stable, it accumulates in animal tissues and in the food chain.

During the 40 years following DDT's commercial introduction in the 1940s, more than 4 billion pounds of it were used to control insect-borne diseases. Until 1972, it was widely used in the United States, mostly on cotton, peanuts, and soybeans. As a result of its use, the residues are now ubiquitous in the environment, and at the present time, some level of DDT can be detected in almost all biological and environmental samples. Because of its high lipid solubility, DDT concentrates in milk. When DDT was in widespread use, levels in human milk and adipose tissue were found to be higher than the concentrations permitted in meat and dairy products; however, since its use has been prohibited, storage levels of DDT in human tissue have declined significantly. DDT is, however, still in use in other countries, largely to control insect-borne diseases that pose a substantial threat to public health.

1. Toxicity

The possible clinical effects of many repeated doses of DDT were first explored in 1945 when a scientist conducted a test, lasting a total of 11.5 months, where he daily inhaled 100 mg of pure DDT and drank water dusted at the rate of 3240 mg/m^2. (See Table 8.3 for acute toxicities.) Much of the inhaled dust must have been deposited in the upper respiratory tract and swallowed. Later, for 1 month he consumed food which

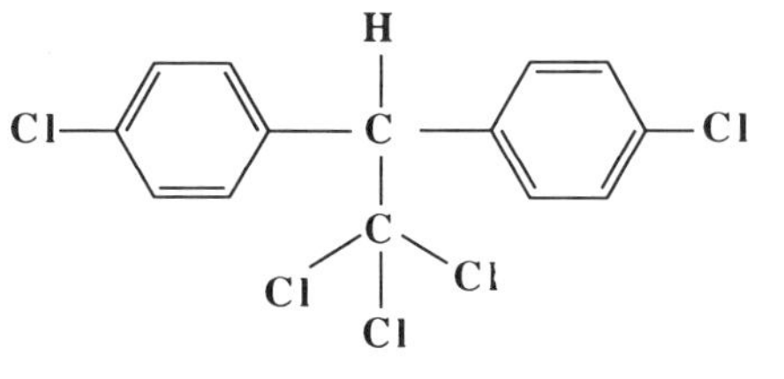

Figure 8.1 Structure of 1,1′-(2,2,2-trichloroethylidene)bis(4-chlorobenzene) (DDT).

TABLE 8.2
Incidence of Malaria before and after the Use of DDT

Country	Year	No. of cases
Cuba	1962	3519
	1969	3
Jamaica	1954	4417
	1969	0
Venezuela	1943	8,171,115
	1958	800
India	1935	>100 million
	1969	285,962
Yugoslavia	1937	169,545
	1969	15
Taiwan	1945	>1 million
	1969	0

had been sprayed with DDT at the rate of 2160 mg/m^2. No ill effect of any kind was observed in either case.

Later studies of DDT in volunteers were designed to explore the details of storage and excretion of the compounds in people and to search for possible effects of doses considered to be safe. In the first of these studies, men were given 0, 3.5, and 35 mg/man/day. These administered dosages, plus DDT measured in the men's food, resulted in dosage levels of 2.1, 3.4, 38, 63, and 610 μg DDT/kg body weight/day.

TABLE 8.3
Acute Oral and Dermal LD_{50} of DDT to Animals

Species	Oral (mg/kg)	Dermal (mg/kg)
Rat	500–2500	1000
Mouse	300–1600	375
Guinea pig	250–560	1000
Rabbit	300–1770	300–2820
Dog	>300	–
Cat	100–410	–

Note. The formulation was water suspension or powder oil solution.

2. In Vivo *Metabolism*

DDT was metabolized to the base-labile glucuronide of bis(*p*-chlorophenyl)acetic acid (DDA) and excreted in urine by Swiss mice and Syrian golden hamsters. The more stable glycine and alanine conjugates of DDA were also found. DDT metabolic intermediate 1-chloro-2,2-bis(*p*-chlorophenyl)ethane (DDMU) is partially metabolized *in vivo* by mice to 2-hydroxy-2,2-bis(*p*-chlorophenyl)acetic acid (OHDDA) and other metabolites that are excreted in urine. The metabolic detoxification sequence of conversion of DDT in rats was shown to be: p,p′-DDT–p,p′-DDE–p,p′-DDMU–p,p′-DDNU–p,p′-DDOH–p,p′-DDA (Figure 8.2).

Oral doses of DDT (5, 10, 20 mg/day) administered to human volunteers were, in part, excreted as DDA. Ingested DDA is promptly and efficiently excreted in the urine, undergoing virtually no tissue storage during ingestion. The results suggest that measurement of urinary DDA excretion offers a useful method of monitoring DDT exposure.

Methoxychlor is a DDT analogue that has replaced DDT in many applications. The structure of methoxychlor is shown in Figure 8.3. Enzymes in both mammals and soil organisms are able to catalyze the demethylation of the methoxy oxygen atoms, producing a more polar degradation product that may be conjugated and excreted. Thus, methoxychlor does not accumulate in animal tissues and does not persist in the environment. Mammalian LD_{50} values for methoxychlor range from 5000 to 6000 mg/kg, 40 to 60 times higher than for DDT. However, methoxychlor also shows less toxicity to its target organisms than does DDT.

B. Chlorinated Cyclodiene Insecticides

Cyclodiene insecticides are an important group of chlorohydrocarbons, most of which are synthesized by the principle of the Diels–Alder reaction. In honor of Alder and Diels, two of the most important representatives are named Aldrin and Dieldrin. The structures of typical cyclodiene insecticides are shown in Figure 8.4. Table 8.4 lists their LD_{50}'s in rats.

1. *Mode of Toxic Action*

Like DDT, these compounds are neurotoxic. However, as a class they are much more toxic to mammals than DDT and tend to produce more severe symptoms, for example, convulsions. The mechanism of neurotoxic action is not understood but is thought to involve disruption of

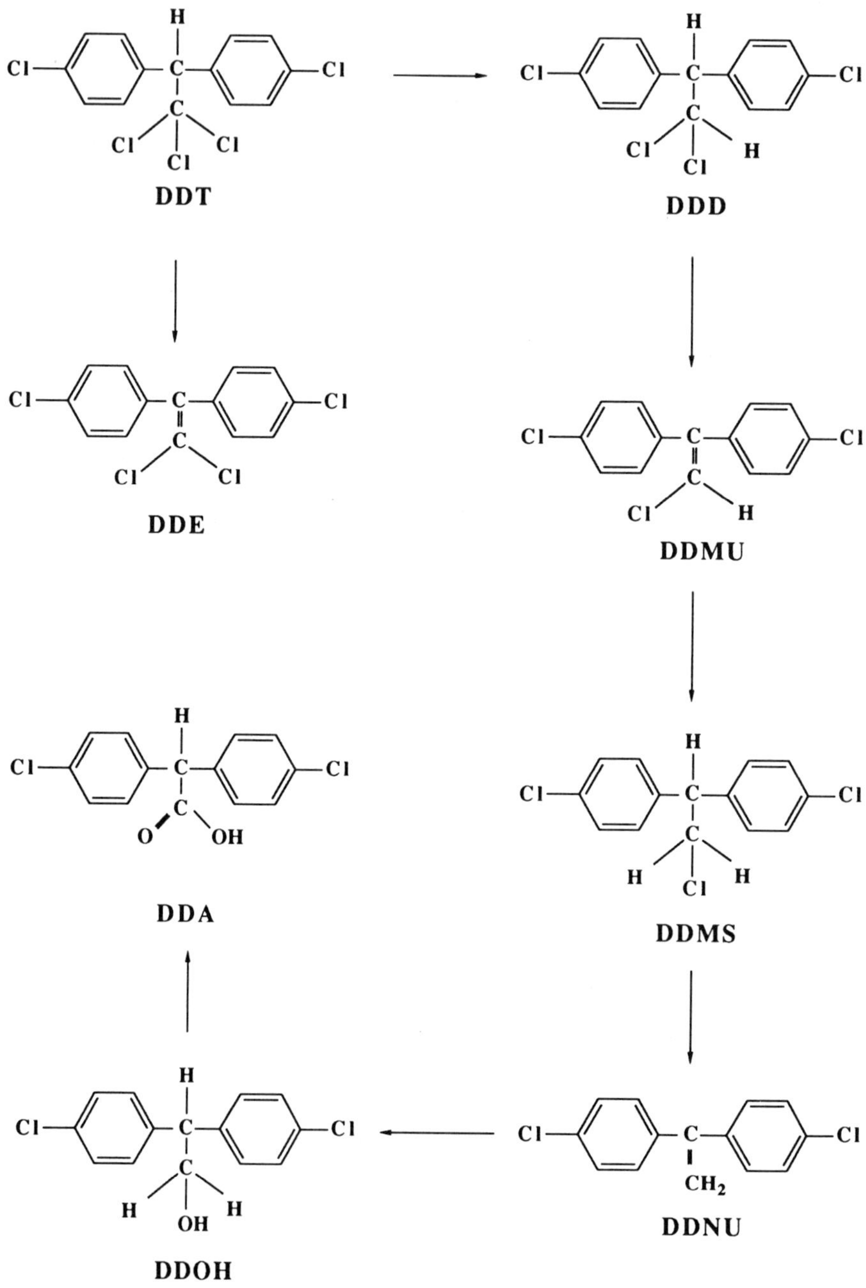

DDT

DDD

DDE

DDMU

DDA

DDMS

DDOH

DDNU

Figure 8.2 Metabolic conversion pathways of DDT.

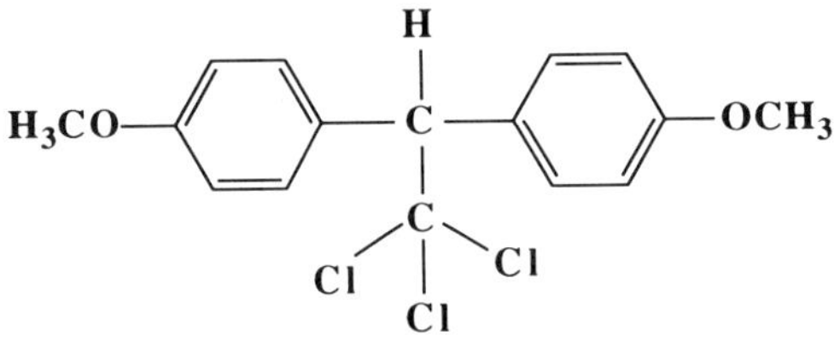

Figure 8.3 Structure of methoxychlor.

nerve impulse transmission by interfering with control of Ca^{2+} and Cl^- concentrations. A number of human poisonings and fatalities have resulted from accidental exposure to Endrin and Dieldrin. Chronic feeding studies in a variety of mammalian species have shown that increased liver weight and histological changes in the liver similar to those caused by DDT are produced by doses of Endrin ranging from 5 to 150 ppm, depending on the species.

Some reproductive toxicity has been reported, but only at doses high enough to cause histological changes in the maternal liver. Many studies of the carcinogenicity of these compounds have been made. Most have

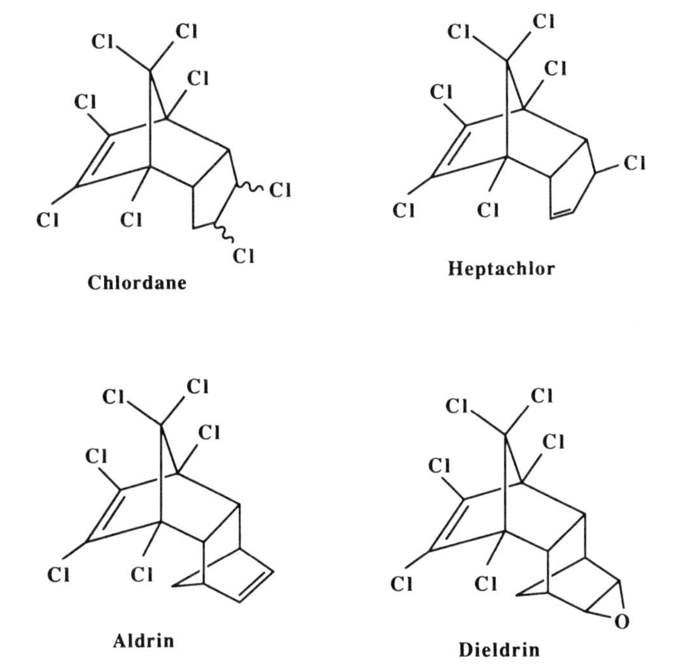

Figure 8.4 Structures of typical cyclodiene insecticides.

TABLE 8.4
LD_{50} (mg/kg) in Rats of Chlorinated Cyclodiene Insecticides

Insecticide	LD_{50}
Chlordane	150–700
Heptachlor	100–163
Aldrin	25–98
Dieldrin	24–98
Endrin	5–43

been inconclusive; however, there is sufficient evidence overall to consider many of these compounds as probable animal carcinogens. Like DDT, these compounds are highly lipid soluble and quite stable. Hence, they accumulate in animal tissues and bioconcentrate in the food chain. As a result, the production and use of these compounds have been sharply reduced, and many have been banned entirely, including Chlordane and Dieldrin.

C. Organophosphate Insecticides

Organophosphate insecticides (OPs) are among the oldest of the synthetic pesticides, and are currently the most widely used class of insecticides. Although Lassaigne first synthesized OPs from the reaction of phosphoric acid with alcohol in 1820, it was not until the 1930s that Schrader discovered their insecticidal properties. At this time, agricultural industry was rapidly expanding and eagerly used synthetic insecticides in addition to such natural insecticides as nicotine, rotenone, and pyrethrum. There are many OPs whose structures are chemically modified. Figure 8.5 shows the structures of some typical OPs. Table 8.5 lists the LD_{50}'s of typical OPs for mice.

1. In Vivo *Metabolism*

The OPs do not accumulate in the body because they are rapidly metabolized and excreted. The OPs also undergo a number of metabolic reactions in mammals. Malathion, for instance, is quite susceptible to hydrolysis by esterases and so has very low mammalian toxicity. Parathion, on the other hand, contains an aromatic phosphate ester group that is more resistant to enzymatic hydrolysis. Activation to its toxic analogue, paraoxon, can thus proceed to a greater extent, resulting in a much

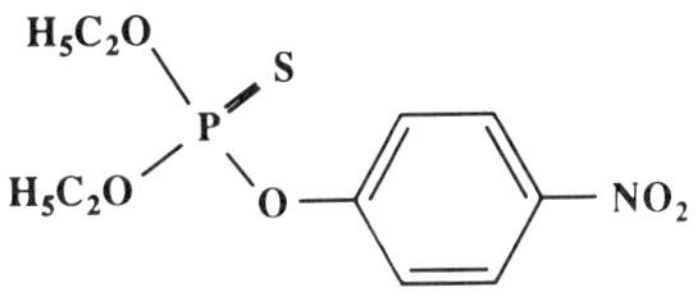

Parathion

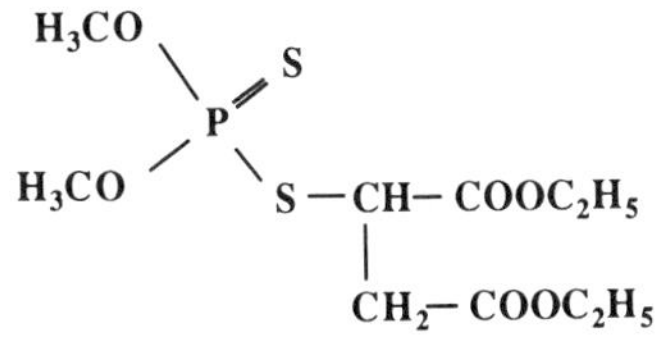

Malathion

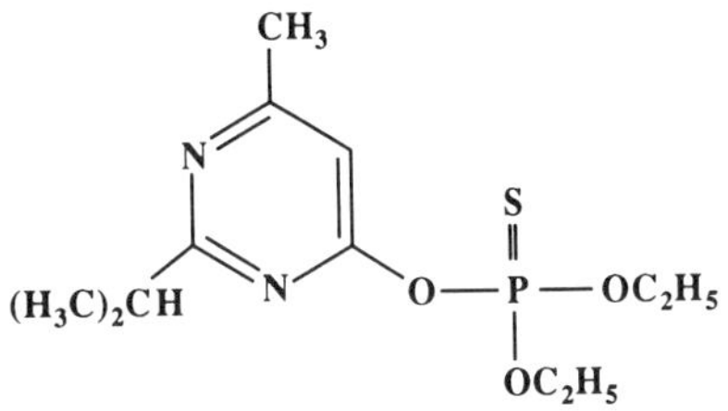

Diazinon

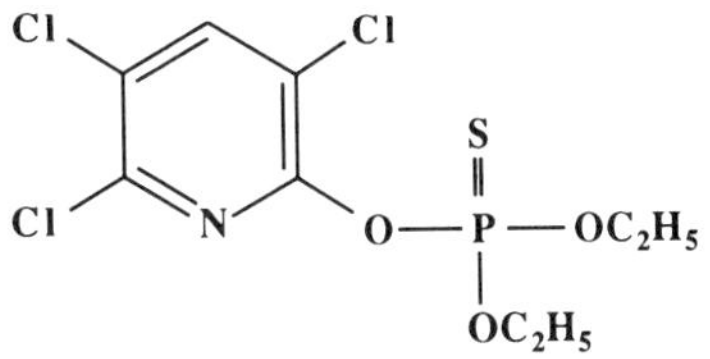

Dursban

Figure 8.5 Structures of typical organophosphate insecticides.

higher mammalian toxicity. Thus, malathion is registered for use by home gardeners, while the use of parathion is restricted to trained applicators. It must be noted that the oxidation of malathion can also occur upon exposure to air. In addition, improper or extended storage can give rise to contamination with the quite toxic malaoxon. Metabolic pathways of OPs are summarized as

1. Oxidation
   - Thiono → oxo-form
   - Oxidative dealkyration
   - Thioether → sulfoxide → sulfone
   - Oxidation of aliphatic substituents
   - Hydroxylation of an aromatic ring

TABLE 8.5
LD_{50} (mg/kg) in Mice of Typical Organophosphate Insecticides

Insecticide	LD_{50}
Parathion	10–12
Methyl parathion	30
Methyl paraoxon	1.4
Paraoxon	0.6–0.8

2. Reduction	Nitro → amino group Other reductions
3. Isomerization	
4. Hydrolysis	Enzymatic Nonenzymatic
5. Dealkylation at the carboxy group	Ester → acid "Saponification"
7. Conjugation	Hydroxy compounds with glucuronic acid Hydroxy compounds with sulfate

2. Mode of Toxic Action

The OPs inhibit activity of acetylcholinesterase (AChE) which is a neurotransmitter in mammals. Normally, acetylcholine (ACh) is rapidly broken down following its release by a group of enzymes known as cholinesterases. OPs, or their metabolites, can compete with acetylcholine for its receptor site on these enzymes, thus blocking the breakdown of ACh. The extent of inhibition of the enzyme depends strongly on steric factors, that is, on how well the inhibitor "fits" on the enzyme, as well as on the nature of the organic groups present. Aromatic groups with electron-withdrawing substituents, as are present in parathion and related compounds, enhance binding to AChE and thus increase toxicity. The resulting accumulation of ACh at smooth muscular junctions causes continued stimulation of the parasympathetic nervous system, producing such symptoms as tightness of the chest, increased salivation, lacrimation, increased sweating, peristalsis (which may lead to nausea, vomiting, cramps, and diarrhea), bradychardia, and a characteristic constriction of the pupils of the eye.

While OPs are a significant occupational hazard to agricultural workers, residues on food products do not normally result in exposures sufficient to lead to toxic symptoms in humans.

D. Carbamate Insecticides

The chemical structures of several important carbamates are shown in Figure 8.6. These compounds are synthetic analogues of the toxic alkaloid physostigimine found in calabar beans. This compound is the toxic principle upon which the "trial-by-poison" of certain West African tribes was based. Related compounds have clinical use in the treatment of glaucoma and other diseases.

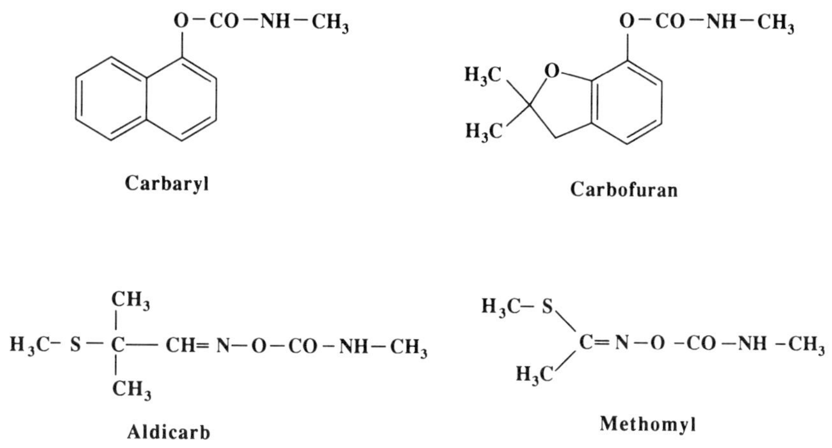

$O-CO-NH-CH_3$

Carbaryl

$O-CO-NH-CH_3$

H_3C O

H_3C

Carbofuran

CH_3

$H_3C-S-C-CH=N-O-CO-NH-CH_3$

CH_3

Aldicarb

H_3C-S

$C=N-O-CO-NH-CH_3$

H_3C

Methomyl

Figure 8.6 Structures of typical carbamate insecticides.

The carbamate insecticides are active against a relatively narrower range of target organisms than the organophosphates, but they are highly toxic to such beneficial insects as honeybees. In general, these compounds are quite toxic to mammals by oral exposure, although in most cases their dermal toxicity is low. Table 8.6 gives the LD_{50}'s in rats for representative carbamate insecticides.

Carbamate insecticides have been involved in a large number of human poisoning incidents, both as a result of occupational exposure and as contamination of food products. For example, the carbamate Aldicarb was the cause of 281 ill in California in 1985 as a result of contaminated watermelons. Because Aldicarb is quite water soluble, it can accumulate to dangerous levels in foods with a high water content. Accordingly, it is not registered for such applications. However, because it is widely used on other crops, the possibility of contamination exists, as shown by the watermelon incident.

TABLE 8.6
LD_{50} (mg/kg) in Rats of Typical Carbamate Insecticides

Insecticide	LD_{50}
Carbaryl	850
Carbofuran	8–14
Aldicarb	0.93
Methomyl	17–24
Aldoxycarb	27

1. *Mode of Toxic Action*

Like the organophosphates, the carbamate insecticides are AChE inhibitors in mammals. The carbamates are direct-acting inhibitors of AChE; however, they are not able to "age" the neurotoxic esterase. Therefore, they are not associated with the delayed neuropathy syndrome. The symptoms of poisoning are typically cholinergic with lacrimation, salivation, miosis, convulsions, and death.

V. Herbicides

The value of harvest losses by pests, diseases, and weeds is estimated worldwide to be about 35% of the potential total harvest. About 9–10% of the reduced yield is caused by weeds. Numerous chemicals have been used as herbicides to prevent weed growth. Consequently, trace amounts of herbicides are present in final food products.

A. Chlorophenoxy Acid Esters

Chlorophenoxy acid esters and their salts are widely used as herbicides. They mimic the plant hormone indole acetic acid and so are able to disrupt the growth of broad-leaf weeds and woody plants. Familiar compounds in this class include 2,4-D and 2,4,5-T (Figure 8.7). These compounds gained considerable notoriety because they were the active ingredients in the defoliant Agent Orange used during the Vietnam War. However, this class of compound has relatively low acute toxicity toward mammals. The acute toxicities (LD_{50}, rat, oral) of 2,4-D and 2,4,5-T are 375 and 500 mg/kg, respectively.

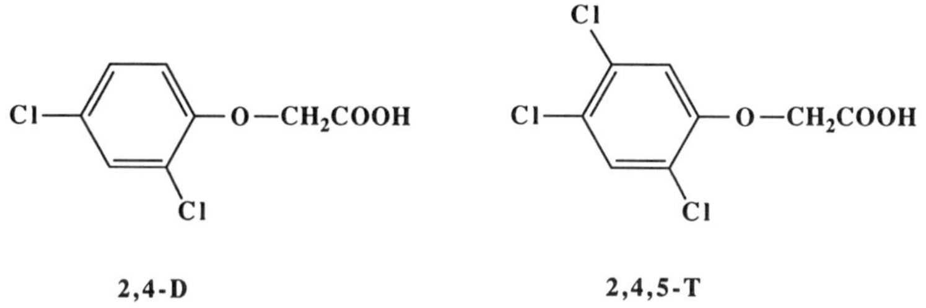

2,4-D 2,4,5-T

Figure 8.7 Structures of typical chlorophenoxy herbicides.

1. Mode of Toxic Action and Toxicity

The mechanisms of mammalian toxicity of chlorophenoxy herbicides are not clear. Sublethal doses cause nonspecific muscle weakness. Higher doses lead progressively to stiffness of the limbs, ataxia, paralysis, and coma. The chlorophenoxy esters are readily hydrolyzed to the acid form. The acids are in some cases sufficiently soluble in water to be excreted directly in urine. In other cases, easily excreted conjugates are formed. Because of the rapid elimination of the acids and conjugates, accumulation in mammalian systems does not occur and chronic effects resulting from low-level exposures are not generally seen.

Formulated chlorophenoxy herbicides have been found to be teratogenic in many animal species. This effect is now thought to be due to a contaminant, TCDD, often referred to as "dioxin" in the popular press. Detains of TCDD are described in Chapter 7.

VI. Naturally Occurring Pesticides

Naturally occurring pesticides have been used in agriculture for a long time. It was recognized early in the 19th century that crushed flowers (pyrethrum powders) from plants in the chrysanthemum family could control insect pests. By 1851, pyrethrum powders were in world wide use. It is now known that at least six active esters are present in pyrethrum, and various synthetic pyrethroids modelled on these natural esters are currently in widespread use. Natural as well as synthetic pyrethroids have very low toxicity to mammals. Nicotine, another natural insecticide, is produced by plants in the tobacco family and was used as an insecticide at least as early as 1763. It is a potent insecticide, with an LD_{50} between 10 and 60 mg/kg for various target species; it also has very high mammalian toxicity by both oral and dermal exposure. Many other plants (walnut trees, for example) secrete chemicals that prevent the growth of competitive plants within their root zone, and thus provide their own pesticide. Finally, the use of various herbs to control particular pests is a recognized part of gardening history, indicating that farmers have accumulated much knowledge regarding the use of chemicals in agriculture.

Suggestions for Further Reading

1. Ayres, J. C., and Kirschman, J. C. (1981). "Impact of Toxicology on Food Processing." AVI Pub. Co., Westport, Connecticut.

2. Duggan, R. E., and Lipscomb, G. Q. (1971). Regulatory control of pesticide residues in foods. *J. Dairy Sci.* **54,** 695.
3. Fennah, R. G. (1945). Preliminary tests with DDT against insect pests of foodcrops in the lesser Antilles. *Trop. Agric.* **22,** 222.
4. Gartrell, M. J., Craun, J. C., Podrebarac, D. S., and Gunderson, E. L. (1985). Pesticides, selected elements, and other chemicals in adult total diet samples, *J. Assoc. Off. Anal. Chem.* **68,** 862.
5. Hathcock, J. N. (ed.) (1982). "Nutritional Toxicology." Academic Press, New York.
6. Pim, L. R. (1981). "The Invisible Additives: Environmental Contaminants in Our Food." Doubleday, Garden City, New Jersey.
7. National Research Council (1987). "Regulating Pesticides in Food: the Delaney Paradox." Committee on Scientific and Regulatory Issues Underlying Pesticide Use Patterns and Agricultural Innovation, Board on Agriculture. National Academy Press, Washington, D.C.
8. Buchel, K. H. (1983). "Chemistry of Pesticides." Wiley, New York.

CHAPTER 9

Food Additives

It is natural for people to desire better foods, not only from the perspective of health but also for taste, color, or texture. Hence, a tremendous number of substances have been used since the beginning of this century to enhance food acceptance.

A food additive is a substance or mixture of substances, other than basic food components, added to food in a scientifically controlled amount. These additions can be made during production, processing, storage, and/or packaging. There are two categories of food additives. The first consists of intentional additives that are purposely added to perform specific functions. They include preservatives, antibacterial agents, bleaching agents, antioxidants, sweeteners, coloring agents, flavoring agents, and nutrient supplements.

Additives of the second type are incidental and may be present in finished food in trace quantities as a result of some phase of production, processing, storage, or packaging. An incidental additive could be a substance present in food due to migration or transfer from the package or processing equipment. Since most food additives are intentionally added substances, only intentional additives are discussed here.

Substances intentionally added to foods vary from preservatives to flavoring materials. Table 9.1 indicates the number of substances used for each purpose to date. Approximately 300 substances are recognized as food additives and 60–70 food additives are ingested daily by every person in the United States Table 9.2 lists the most common food additives used for various purposes.

Despite the fact that food additives undergo extensive laboratory testing before they are put into commercial food products, the use of additives in foods has engendered great controversy and widespread public concern. There are two basic positions concerning the use of food

TABLE 9.1
Approximate Number of Different Types of Food Additives

Purpose of additive	Number of different additives
Preservatives	30
Antioxidants	28
Sequestrants	44
Surfactants	85
Stabilizers	31
Bleaching, maturing agents	24
Buffers, acids, alkalies	60
Coloring agents	35
Special sweeteners	9
Nutrient supplements	>100
Flavoring agents	>700
Natural flavoring materials	>350

additives. One is that all additives are potential health threats and should not, on that basis, be used. The other is that unless an additive is proved to be hazardous, using it to protect food from spoilage or to increase its nutritional completeness, palatability, texture, or appearance is well justified. The former opinion has been voiced by some consumers. Their concern is that basic food materials are already contaminated by many toxic substances such as pesticides and microorganisms. Once additives are approved for use in a food product, people will be ingesting them continuously. Therefore, even when an acceptable daily intake (ADI) has been officially established and each product remains within those limits, total ingestion of certain additives from various sources may exceed the

TABLE 9.2
The Most Common Chemicals Developed as Food Additives

Purposes	Chemicals
Preservative	Benzoic acid, sorbic acid, *p*-oxybenzoic acid, salicylic acid, hydrogen peroxide, AF-2[a]
Antioxidants	Ascorbic acid, DL-α-tocopherol, BHA, propyl gallate
Sweeteners	Saccharine, dulcin, sodium cyclamate[a]
Coloring agents	Food Red No. 2,[a] Food Yellow No. 4, Scarlet Red, Indigo–carmine
Flavoring agents	Safrole,[a] methyl anthranilate, maltol, carvone
Bleaching agents	$CaOCl_2$, NaOCl, $NaClO_2$, SO_2
Nutrient supplements	Vitamins

[a] Banned for use in food.

ADI. This position holds that the chronic toxicities, such as carcinogenicity and teratogenicity, of food additives have not yet been sufficiently studied. In fact, most food additives are used without any information being made available to consumers about their chronic toxicities. Due to the high costs of testing and other factors, progress in research on the chronic toxicities of food additives is very slow.

The second basic position regarding food additives points out their many benefits: Were it not for food additives, baked goods would go stale or mold overnight, salad oils and dressings would separate and turn rancid, table salt would turn hard and lumpy, canned fruits and vegetables would become discolored or mushy, vitamin potencies would deteriorate, beverages and frozen desserts would lack flavor, and wrappings would stick to the contents.

Within the current structure of the food processing industry in the United States, it would be virtually impossible to abandon food additives entirely. However, in order to provide the maximum protection to the consumers, it is wise to study any potential toxicity of the food additives in current use.

I. Regulations

The quality of the food supply in the United States is regulated by numerous state and federal laws. Before the turn of the century, most states had laws that protected consumers from hazardous or improperly processed foods, but there was no corresponding federal regulatory framework. Public sentiment became focused on the wholesomeness of the food supply following the publication of Upton Sinclair's novel, *The Jungle,* in which the deplorable conditions in slaughter houses was described. In addition, Dr. Harvey W. Wiley, who was a chemist in the U.S. Department of Agriculture from 1883 to 1930, began conducting chemical and biological analyses of substances in food and discovered instances of misbranded and adulterated food. Since colonies of experimental animals had not yet been developed, Wiley conducted biological testing on himself and a group of young men, who became known as the poison squad. Because of the work of Wiley and his group, reliable information on the adulteration, toxicity, and misbranding of food was obtained. The Pure Food and Drug Act was finally passed in 1906 after years of effort to enact such a law. However, it has been suggested that it passed only because it was presented along with the Meat Inspection Act, a response to the public outcry engendered by Upton Sinclair's novel.

The 1906 Pure Food and Drug Act forbade the production of misbranded and adulterated food products in the District of Columbia and prohibited interstate distribution of fraudulent and unhealthy products. It banished such chemical preservatives as boric acid, salicylic acid, and formaldehyde; additionally, it defined food adulteration as the addition of poisons and deleterious materials, the extraction of valuable constituents and the concealment of the resulting inferiority, substitution of other constituents, and the mixture of substances that would adversely affect health.

The next major piece of legislation was the Federal Food, Drug, and Cosmetic Act of 1938, which added further provisions to the 1906 legislation. It defined food as

1. substances used as food or drink by people or animals,
2. chewing gum, and
3. substances used for components of any such food material.

The law also established standards of product identity and fill, prohibited adulteration, mandated truthful labeling, and restricted the use of chemicals to those required in the manufacturing of the food, with specific tolerance levels set for chemicals with appreciable toxicity.

The Food Additive Amendment that was added to the law in 1958 had a great impact on the food manufacturing industry. While this amendment to the 1938 Act gave official recognition of the U.S. government's tolerance regarding the use of food additives and acceptance of the necessity of additives for a wholesome and abundant food supply, it also took the government out of the business of toxicity testing. The amendment stipulated that any food additive was to be proven safe by the manufacturer, who must also prove toxicity. Thus, the additive manufacturer was requested to bear the burden of lengthy delays in production and the cost of the millions of dollars required for such testing.

The amendment, however, did not apply to additives in use prior to 1958. The potential hazards of these substances were initially assessed based on the opinions of specialists working in the general field of toxicology. Those substances that were considered unsafe for general use in foods were prohibited from further use or strict limits were placed on the levels that could be added to foods. Those substances for which no concerns were expressed were considered "generally recognized as safe" (GRAS). Substances on the GRAS list can be used by manufacturers within the general tenets of good manufacturing practices.

Also included in the Food Additive Amendment of 1958 was the

Delaney clause, which was proposed in response to the increasing concern over the possible role of food additives in human cancer. It states that no substance shall be added to food if it is found by proper testing to cause cancer in people or animals. Although the Delaney clause seems to be a very straightforward and simple way of handling a potentially dangerous class of substances, it provides little room for scientific interpretation of data and remains controversial. The Delaney clause gives no consideration to the specific dose of a substance likely to be encountered in foods and there is no provision for interpretation of animal results in terms of the site of carcinogenesis, known sensitivity of the experimental model, or the specific dose of carcinogens required to produce the cancer. Although several substances have been banned from food use because of apparent carcinogenicity, in no case has the Delaney clause been invoked. All substances banned from use have been banned under the general safety provisions of the 1938 act.

The Color Additive Amendments of 1960 took special notice of color additives and their potential for misuse and toxicity. These amendments differentiated between natural and synthetic color additives and required

1. listing of all color additives on labels;
2. certification of batches of listed colors where this was deemed necessary to protect public health;
3. retesting for safety of previously certified colors using modern techniques and procedures where any questions of safety had arisen since the original listing of the color as safe; and
4. testing of all color additives for food in long-term dietary studies that included carcinogenesis and teratogenesis studies in two or more animal species.

There are currently two classifications considered suitable for use in food colors, GRAS colors and certified colors. GRAS colors are generally pigments that occur naturally in plants and animals or that are simple organic or inorganic compounds; they are exempt from the certification procedure required for most of the synthetic colors. In order to be certified, a sample of each batch of a color must be submitted to the FDA for analyses. The batch receives approval for use if the sample meets previously established standards of quality. Each batch must be analyzed to ensure that the chemical compositions in the new batches are the same as the composition of the batch that was subjected to biological testing.

The practice of periodic review is now also used for all food additives. Since 1970 the FDA has been reviewing GRAS substances and ingredients with prior sanctions according to current standards of safety. Under the current regulatory framework, no substance that appears directly or indirectly in the food may be added to or used on or near food, unless

1. the substance is GRAS,
2. the substance has been granted prior sanction or approval, or
3. a food additive regulation has been issued establishing the conditions for its safe use.

All non-flavor substances on the GRAS list are under review individually in accordance with present-day safety standards while all of the roughly 1000 flavoring agents used in food are reevaluated under a separate program that considers these substances by chemical class. After a GRAS review is completed, a substance with previous GRAS status will be

1. reaffirmed as GRAS;
2. classified as a food additive and conditions of use, levels of use, and any other limitations will be specified;
3. placed under an interim food additive regulation, which indicates that further toxicological information must be obtained for the substance; or
4. prohibited from use.

Substances in the interim food additive category can be used in foods while the testing is going on if there is no undue risk to the public. A substance with GRAS status has no specific quantitative limitations on its use; however, its use is restricted by general definitions of adulterated food as specified in the 1938 Act and by what is designated good manufacturing practice (GMP). GMP includes the following conditions for substances added to food:

1. the quantity of a substance added to food does not exceed the amount reasonably required to accomplish its intended physical, nutritional, or other technical effect in food; and
2. the quantity of a substance that becomes a component of food as a result of its use in the manufacturing, processing, or packaging of food in which it is not intended to accomplish any physical or other technical effect in the food itself shall be reduced to the extent reasonably possible.

GMP also specified that the substance is of appropriate food grade and is prepared and handled as a food ingredient.

Generally, food additives are regulated in amendments under Section 409 of the Food, Drug, and Cosmetic Act of 1938. The law requires not only that food additives be safe at the levels used, but also effective in accomplishing their intended effect. Ineffective additives cannot legally be used regardless of their safety. However, this law specifically excludes certain classes of compounds. Pesticide residues in raw agricultural products are not legally considered to be food additives in the United States, although they are subject to regulation by the EPA and the individual states. Colorants are regulated separately under the Color Additive Amendments to the FD&C Act in 1960.

Prior to the 1958 food additive amendments to the FD&C act, most food additives were not regulated directly, although certain individual substances were banned by the FDA. Additives that were in common and widespread use in 1958 were exempted from requirements of safety testing on the basis of the long experience with these compounds. They were termed GRAS under conditions of their intended use, usually at the lowest practical level and in accordance with good manufacturing practices. Although the FDA has specifically listed hundreds of additives as GRAS, the published list is not inclusive.

II. Preservatives

The development of methods of food preservation was essential to the prehistoric transition of humans from nomadic hunter–gatherer tribes to settled agricultural communities. One of the most important functions of food additives is to preserve food products from spoilage. Since the dawn of history, people have had a great struggle to preserve enough food to survive from one growing season to the next. Even at the present time, it is estimated that up to one-third of the agricultural production of the United States is lost after harvest. Much of this loss results from microbial action or oxidation. Preservatives prevent the spoilage of foods caused by the action of microorganisms.

Smoke was probably the first preservative agent to be discovered. Common salt was also used in prehistoric times. Ancient Egyptians made use of vinegar, oil, and honey, substances that still find application today. The use of sulfur dioxide as a fumigant was described in ancient Assyria, Greece, and China. By the late Middle Ages, it was widely used throughout Europe for preserving wine and possibly had other applications as well. In what may have been the first legal actions directed against chemical food additives, a number of decrees were promulgated to regulate the use of sulfur in wine production during the late 15th century. Pickling was invented by Beukels in the 13th century. No other chemical preservatives were introduced until the late 18th century when Hofer suggested that borax (hydrated sodium borate) be used.

Synthetic chemicals began to be used as food preservatives at the beginning of 20th century, and the widespread use of these chemicals made a wider variety of food available for longer periods of time to more people.

There are many criticisms of the use of food preservatives. However, the considerable time between the production and the consumption of food today makes some use of preservatives necessary in order to prevent spoilage and undesirable alterations in color and flavor. Many microorganisms, including yeasts, molds, and bacteria, can produce undesirable effects in the appearance, taste, or nutritional value of foods. A number of these organisms produce toxins that pose high risks to human health. Atmospheric oxygen can also adversely affect foods, as for example in the development of rancidity in fats.

The word *preservative* has gradually been given broader connotation, covering not only compounds that suppress microbes but also compounds that prevent chemical and biochemical deterioration. The action of preservatives is not to kill bacteria (bactericidal) but rather to delay their action by suppressing their activity (bacteriastatic).

Before being considered for use in food, a chemical preservative must fulfill certain conditions, such as

1. it must be nontoxic and suitable for application,
2. it must not impart off-flavors when used at levels effective in controlling microbial growth,
3. it must be readily soluble,
4. it must exhibit anti-microbial properties over the pH range of each particular food, and
5. it should be economical and practical to use.

A. Benzoic Acid

Benzoic acid, which is usually used in the form of its sodium salt, sodium benzoate (Figure 9.1), has long been used as an antimicrobial additive in foods. It is used in carbonated and still beverages, syrups, fruit salads, icings, jams, jellies, preserves, salted margarine, mincemeat, pickles and relishes, pie, pastry fillings, prepared salads, fruit cocktail, soy sauce, and caviar. The use level ranges from 0.05 to 0.1%.

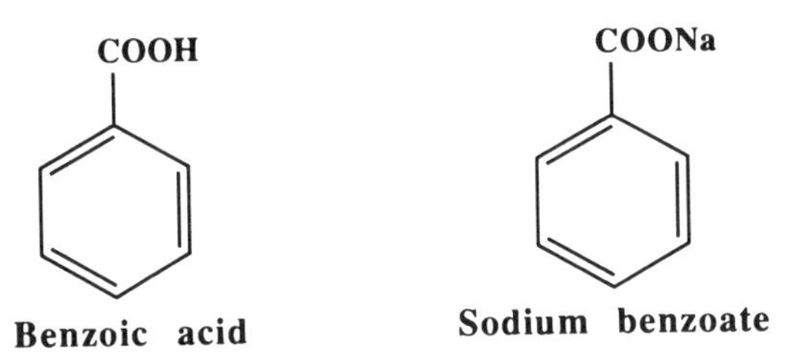

Figure 9.1 Structures of benzoic acid and sodium benzoate.

Benzoic acid in the acid form is quite toxic but its sodium salt is much less toxic (Table 9.3). The sodium salt is preferred because of the low aqueous solubility of the free acid. *In vivo,* the salt is converted to acid, which is the more toxic form.

Studies of the subacute toxicity of benzoic acid in mice indicated that ingestion of benzoic acid or its sodium salt caused weight loss, diarrhea, irritation of internal membranes, internal bleeding, enlargement of liver and kidney, hypersensitivity, and paralysis followed by death. When benzoic acid (80 mg/kg body weight) and sodium bisulfate (160 mg/kg body weight) or their mixture (benzoic acid/sodim bisulfate = 80 mg/160 mg) were fed to mice for 10 weeks, the death rate was 66% from the mixture and 32% from benzoic acid alone.

Chronic toxicities were examined using diets containing 0, 0.5, and 1% of benzoic acid that were fed to male and female rats kept together for 8 weeks. The second generation was observed through its entire life cycle and the third and fourth generations were examined by autopsy. No changes in normal patterns of growth, reproduction, or lactation during life were recorded and no morphological abnormalities were observed from the autopsies.

Degradation pathways for benzoic acid have also been studied in detail and the results have supported harmlessness of this substance. The metabolic breakdown pathways of benzoic acid are shown in Figure 9.2.

TABLE 9.3
Acute Toxicity of Sodium Benzoate

Animal	Method	LD_{50} (mg/kg)
Rat	Oral	2700
Rat	Intravenous injection	1714 ± 124
Rabbit	Oral	2000
Rabbit	Subcutaneous injection	2000
Dog	Oral	2000

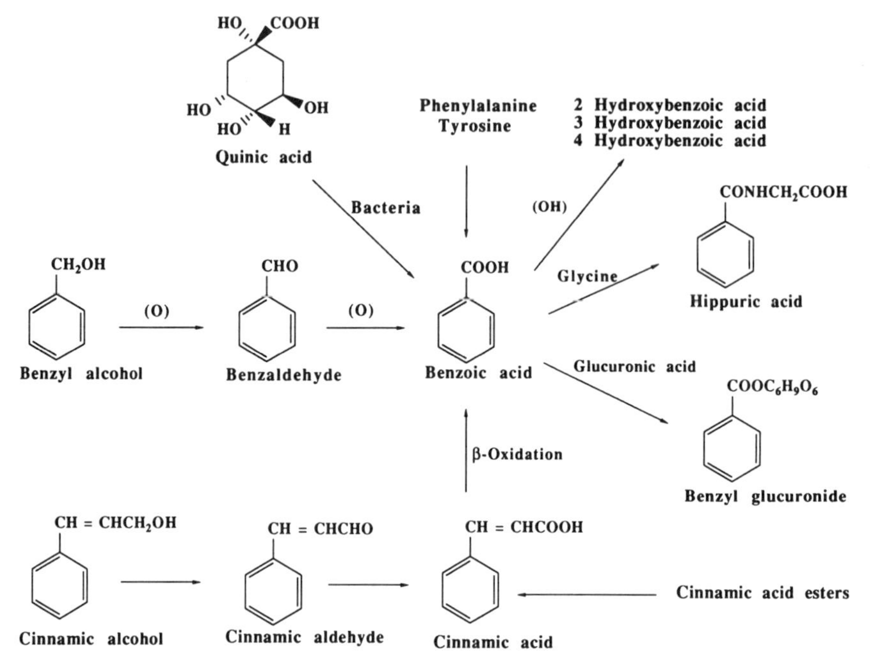

Figure 9.2 The metabolic breakdown pathways of benzoic acid.

The total dose of benzoic acid is excreted within 10–14 hr and 75–80% is excreted within 6 hr. After conjugation with glycine, 90% of benzoic acid appears in the urine as hippuric acid. The rest forms a glucuronide, 1-benzoylglucuronic acid. The lower aliphatic esters of benzoic acid are first hydrolyzed by esterase, which abounds in the intestinal wall and liver. The resulting benzoic acid is subsequently degraded in the usual manner.

B. Sorbic Acid and Potassium Sorbate

Sorbic acid and its salts have broad-spectrum activity against yeast and molds, but are less active against bacteria. The antimicrobial action of sorbic acid was independently discovered in the United States and Germany in 1939, and since the mid-1950s sorbates have been increasingly used as preservatives. The structures of these compounds are shown in Figure 9.3. The sorbates have generally been found superior to benzoate for preservation of margarine, fish, cheese, bread, and cake. Sorbic acid and its potassium salts are used in low concentrations to control mold

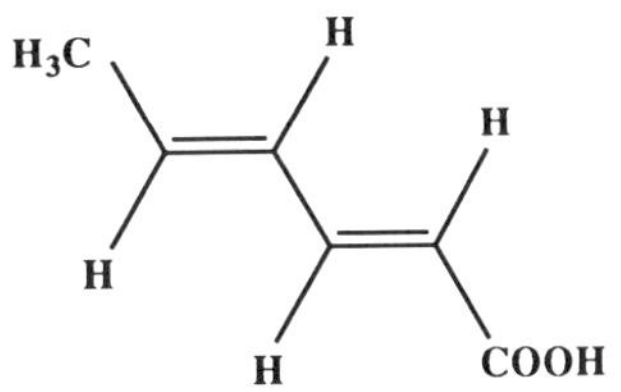

Sorbic acid 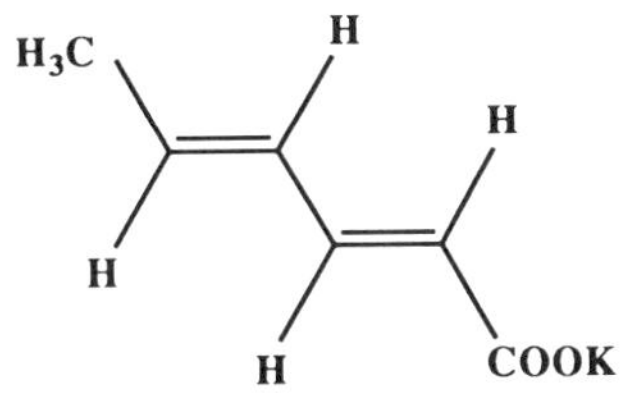 **Potassium sorbate**

Figure 9.3 Structures of sorbic acid and postassium sorbate.

and yeast growth in cheese products, baked foods, fruit beverages, pickles, fresh fruits and vegetables, some fish and meat products, and wines.

Sorbic acid is practically nontoxic. Table 9.4 shows acute toxicity of sorbic acid and its potassium salt. Animal studies have not shown obvious problems even in tests performed with large doses for longer time periods. When sorbic acid (40 mg/kg/day) was injected directly into the stomach of male and female mice for 2 months, no differences were observed in survival rates, growth rates, or appetite between the injected mice and the controls. When the dose was increased to 80 mg/kg/day for 3 additional months, however, some growth inhibition was observed. When potassium sorbate (1 and 2% in feed) was fed to dogs for 3 months, no pathological abnormalities were observed. This evidence indicates that the subacute toxicity of sorbic acid is negligible.

Chronic toxicities of sorbic acid using various animals have shown that neither sorbic acid nor its potassium salt induces malignant growths in animals. For example, rats fed with 5% sorbic acid in feed for two generations (1000 days) showed no changes in growth rates, rates of reproduction, or any other behaviors.

As a relatively new food additive, sorbate has been subject to stringent

TABLE 9.4
Acute Toxicity of Sorbic Acid and Its Potassium Salt

Animal	Compound	Method	LD_{50} (g/kg)
Rat	Sorbic acid	Oral	10.5
Rat	Potassium sorbate	Oral	4.2
Mouse	Sorbic acid	Oral	>8
Mouse	Potassium sorbate	Oral	4.2
Mouse	Sorbic acid	ip	2.8
Mouse	Potassium sorbate	ip	1.3

toxicity-testing requirements. It may well be the most intensively studied of all chemical food preservatives. In 90-day feeding studies in rats and dogs and a lifetime feeding study in rats, a 5% dietary level of sorbates produced no observable adverse effects. At a 10% level in a 120-day feeding study, rats showed increased growth and increased liver weight. This has been attributed to the caloric value of sorbate at these high dietary levels since it can act as a substrate for normal catabolic metabolism in mammals. No reproductive toxicity has been observed and sorbates are not mutagenic or tumoregenic.

C. Hydrogen Peroxide

Hydrogen peroxide has been used in the dairy industry as a substitute for heat pasteurization in the treatment of milk and as a direct preservative to improve the keeping quality. It also has a bleaching effect, and in Japan it has been used as a preservative for fish-paste products. The use of highly pure hydrogen peroxide in manufactured cheese has been approved by the United States Food and Drug Administration (industrial grade hydrogen peroxide is usually a 3–35% aqueous solution; a commercial home product is a 3% aqueous solution).

Acute toxicities (LD_{50}) of hydrogen peroxide for rat are 700 mg/kg/bw and 21 mg/kg/bw by subcutaneous injection and intravenous injection, respectively. When large amounts of hydrogen peroxide were injected directly into the stomachs of rats, weight and blood protein concentrations were changed slightly. When hydrogen peroxide was mixed with feed, however, no abnormalities were observed. While the use of bactericides has been limited due to their toxicity to humans, only hydrogen peroxide is currently recognized for use.

D. AF-2 [2-(2-Furyl)-3-(5-nitro-2-furyl)acrylamide]

The antibacterial activity of nitrofuran derivatives was first recognized in 1944. The disclosed antibacterial properties of these compounds had created a new group of antimicrobial agents. Such activity is dependent on the presence of a nitro group in the 5-position of the furan ring. Numerous 5-nitrofuran derivatives have been synthesized and certain compounds have been widely used in clinical and veterinary medicine and as antiseptics for animal feeds.

AF-2 (Figure 9.4) was legally approved for use in Japan in 1965 and was added to soybean curd (tofu), ham, sausage, fish ham, fish sausage,

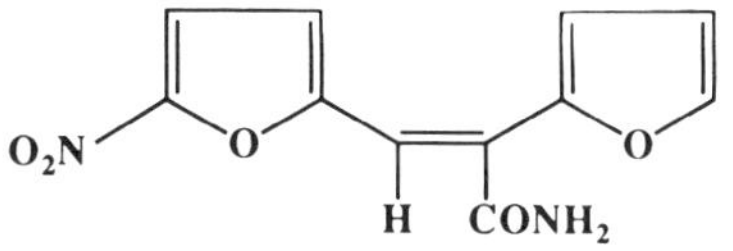

Figure 9.4 Structure of 2-(2-furyl)-3-(5-nitro-2-furyl)acrylamide (AF-2).

and fish paste (kamaboko). The safety-testing data on which the compound was approved were those obtained for acute and chronic toxicity for 2 years and reproductive potential for four generations using mice and rats. At the time, no attention was paid to mutagenicity. In 1973, AF-2 was proved to be mutagenic in various microbial test systems. The mutagenicity of this food additive strongly suggested its carcinogenicity and the risk of its use as a food additive. Within 1 or 2 years after the discovery of its mutagenicity, the actual carcinogenicity of this chemical was demonstrated in animal studies. Since that time, more emphasis has been place on finding causative agents of cancer.

Short-term bioassays had received much attention because they were able to screen suspected carcinogens. The mechanism of carcinogenesis is not yet clear, but a close relation between carcinogens and mutagens has been demonstrated. AF-2 was the first example of a compound that was shown to be a carcinogen. The fact that AF-2 was discovered first to be mutagenic proved the value of mutagenicity testing as a screening method for carcinogens.

III. Antioxidants

One of the most common types of food deteriorations is an undesirable change in color or flavor caused by oxygen in air (oxidative deterioration). Oxidation causes changes not only in color or flavor but also decreases the nutritional value of food and sometimes produces toxic materials. Most foods consist mainly of carbohydrates, fats, proteins, and water. While microbiological spoilage is one of the most important factors to be considered in preserving carbohydrate and protein portions of food products, oxidation (particularly atmospheric oxidation) is the chief factor in degradation of fats and fatty portions of foods. Oxidative deterioration of fat results not only in the destruction of vitamins A, D, E, K, and C, but also in the destruction of essential fatty acids and the development of a pungent and offensive off-flavor. In extreme cases, toxic by-products have resulted from oxidative reactions.

The most efficient method to prevent oxidative degradation is the use of antioxidative agents. The antioxidants may be classed as natural and synthetic. Naturally occurring antioxidants exhibit relatively weak antioxidant properties. As a consequence, synthetic antioxidants have been developed for use in foods. In order for these substances to be allowed in foods, they must have a low toxicity; should be effective in low concentrations in a wide variety of fats; should contribute no objectionable flavor, odor, or color to the product; and should have approval by the Food and Drug Administration.

A. L-Ascorbic Acid (Vitamin C)

L-Ascorbic acid, or vitamin C, is widely present in plants. The structures of ascorbic acid and dehydroascorbic acid are shown in Figure 9.5. Vitamin C is not only an important nutrient but is also used as an antioxidant in various foods. However, it is not soluble in fat and is unstable under basic conditions. Vitamin C reduces cadmium toxicity and excess doses prolong the retention time of an organic mercury compound in a biological system. Overdoses of vitamin C (106 g) induce perspiration, nervous tension, and lowered pulse rate. WHO recommends that daily intake be less than 0.25 mg/kg. Toxicity due to ascorbic acid has not been reported. Although repeated intravenous injections of 80 mg dehydroascorbic acid was reported to be diabetogenic in rats, oral consumption of 1.5 g/day of ascorbic acid for 6 weeks had no effect on glucose tolerance or glycosuria in 12 normal adult males and produced no change in blood glucose concentrations in 80 diabetics after 5 days. The same report noted that a 100-mg intravenous dose of dehydroascorbic acid given daily for pro-

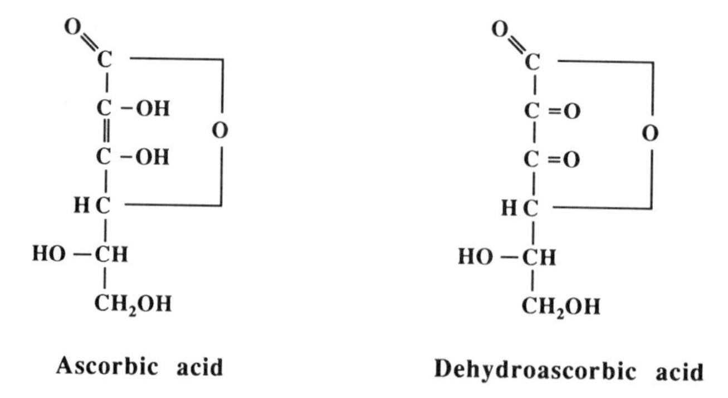

Figure 9.5 Structures of ascorbic acid and dehydroascorbic acid.

longed periods produced no signs of diabetes. Ascorbic acid is readily oxidized to dehydroascorbic acid, which is reduced by glutathione in blood.

B. dl-α-Tocopherol (Vitamin E)

α-Tocopherol is known as vitamin E and exists in many kind of plants, especially in lettuce and alfalfa. Its color changes from yellow to dark brown when exposed to sunlight. The structure of α-tocopherol is shown in Figure 9.6.

Natural vegetable oils are not readily oxidized due to the presence of tocopherol. During refining processes, however, tocopherol may be removed from oils; consequently, refined vegetable oils can become unstable toward oxidation. In one experiment, vitamin E appeared to be relatively innocuous, having been given to patients for months both orally and parenterally at a dosage level of 300 mg/day without any observed ill effects. However, in another experiment, 6 out of 13 patients given similar doses complained of headache, nausea, fatigue, dizziness, and blurred vision.

Although the chronic toxicity of vitamin E has not been thoroughly studied, WHO recommends 2 mg/kg/day as the maximum daily dose.

C. Propyl Gallate

Propyl gallate (*n*-propyl-3,4,5-trihydroxybenzoate, Figure 9.7) is used in vegetable oils and butter. When 1.2 or 2.3% propyl gallate was added to feed for rats, loss of weight was observed. This may be due to the rats' reluctance to eat food which was contaminated with the bitter taste of propyl gallate. When it was given for 10–16 months at the 2–3% level, 40% of the rats died within the first month and the remainder showed severe growth inhibition. Autopsies of rats indicated kidney damage re-

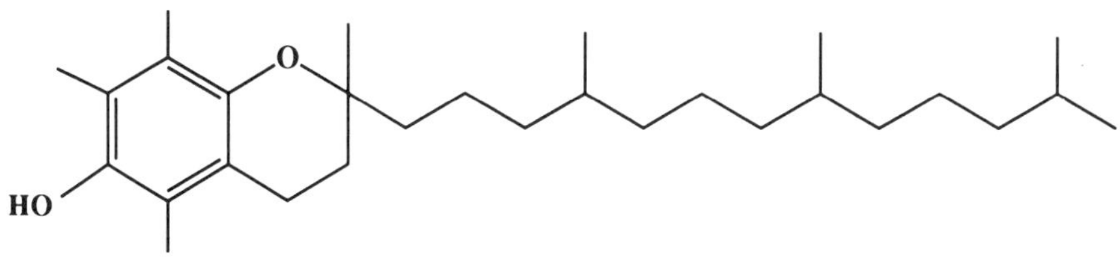

Figure 9.6 Structure of α-tocopherol (vitamin E).

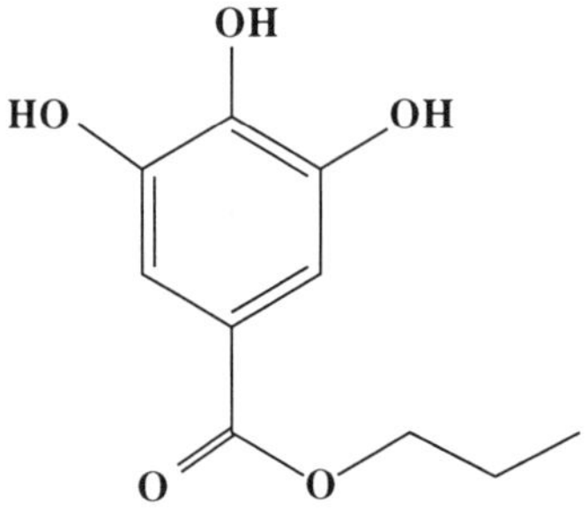

Figure 9.7 Structure of *n*-propyl-3,4,5-trihydroxybenzoate (propyl gallate).

sulting from the ingestion of propyl gallate. However, no other animal studies show serious problems and further studies indicated that propyl gallate does not cause serious chronic toxicities.

D. Butylated Hydroxyanisole and Butylated Hydroxytoluene

Butylated hydroxyanisole (BHA) and butylated hydroxytoluene (BHT) are the most commonly used antioxidants and present constant intractable problems to the food industry. The structures of BHA and BHT are shown in Figure 9.8.

BHA produces mild diarrhea in dogs when it is fed continuously for 4 weeks at the level of 1.4–4.7 g/kg. It also causes chronic allergic reactions, malformations, and damage to the metabolic system. When BHT was fed to rats at levels of 0.2, 0.5, and 0.8% mixed with feed for 24 months, no

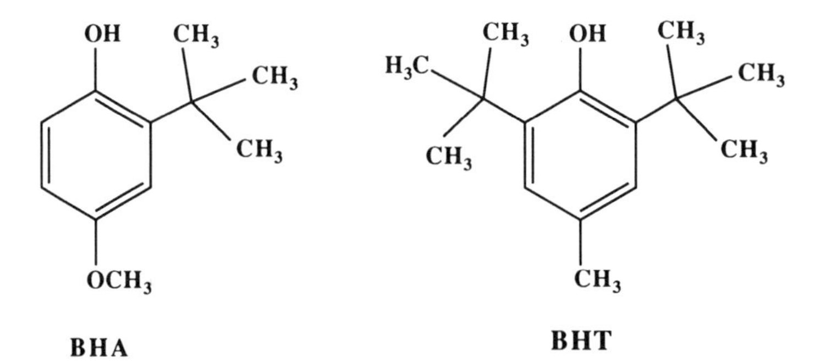

Figure 9.8 Structures of butylated hydroxyanisole (BHA) and butylated hydroxytoluene (BHT).

pathological changes were observed. The some results were obtained when the dose was increased to 1% of the feed.

Antioxidants—including vitamin C, vitamin E, BHA, and BHT—have some anticarcinogenic activities. They have been used to study mechanisms of chemical carcinogenesis. If BHT is mixed with a known carcinogen such as N-2-fluorenyl acetamide (FAA) or azoxymethane in the feed, the rate of tumor induction in rats is diminished. The mechanisms of antioxidants in chemical carcinogenesis are not well understood yet, but the relationship between chemical carcinogens and BHT has been intensively investigated.

IV. Sweeteners

Naturally occurring sweeteners such as honey and sucrose were known to the ancient Romans. However, sweeteners obtained from natural sources have been limited. To supplement the demand, sweetening agents such as saccharin have been synthesized since the late 19th century. Recently, these non-nutritive sweeteners have begun to receive much attention as ingredients in low-calorie soft drinks. The synthetic, or non-carbohydrate, sweeteners provide sweetened foods for diabetics who must limit sugar intake, for those who wish to limit carbohydrate calorie intake, and for those who desire to reduce food-induced dental caries.

A. Saccharin and Sodium Saccharin

Saccharin, which is 300–500 times sweeter than sucrose, is one of the most commonly used artificial sweeteners. The name saccharin is a commercial name of Fahlberg and List Company. The sodium salt is the form actually used in the formulation of foods and beverages (Figure 9.9). Its acute toxicity is shown in Table 9.5.

It has been questioned whether or not saccharin is a health hazard. In 1972, it was found that 7.5% of saccharin in feed produced bladder cancer in the second generation of rats. Some reports, however, showed contradictory results. Consequently, WHO has recommended that daily intake of saccharin be limited to 0–0.5 mg/kg. The carcinogenicity of saccharin is still under investigation. When pellets of saccharin and cholesterol (1:4) were placed in the bladders of mice, tumors developed after 40–52 weeks.

When 2.6 g/kg of a mixture of sodium cyclamate and saccharin (10:1)

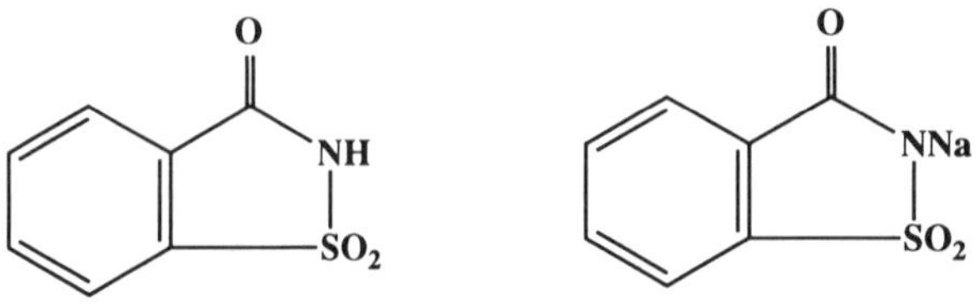

Saccharin Sodium saccharin

Figure 9.9 Structures of saccharin and sodium saccharin.

was given to rats for 80 days, eight rats developed bladder tumors after 105 weeks. When only sodium cyclamate was fed for 2 years, bladder cancer also appeared. The main attention has, therefore, been given to the carcinogenicity of sodium cyclamate.

B. Sodium Cyclamate

Sodium cyclamate is an odorless, white crystalline powder. It is about 30 times as sweet as sucrose in dilute solution. The structure of sodium cyclamate is shown in Figure 9.10 and its acute toxicity is shown in Table 9.6.

Capillary transitional cell tumors were found in the urinary bladders of 8 out of 80 rats that received 2600 mg/kg of body weight per day of a mixture of sodium cyclamate and sodium saccharin (10:1) for up to 105 weeks. When the test mixture was fed at dietary levels designed to furnish 500, 1120, and 2500 mg/kg body weight to groups of 35 and 45 female rats, the only significant finding was the occurrence of papillar carcinomas in the bladders of 12 of 70 rats fed the maximum dietary level of the mixture (equivalent to about 25 g/kg body weight) for periods ranging

TABLE 9.5
Acute Toxicity of Sodium Saccharin

Animal	Method	LD_{50} (g/kg)
Mouse	Oral	17.5
Mouse	ip	6.3
Rat (mongrel)	Oral	17.0
Rat (mongrel)	ip	7.1
Rat (Wistar)	Oral	14.2 ± 1.3
Rabbit	Oral	5–8 (LD)

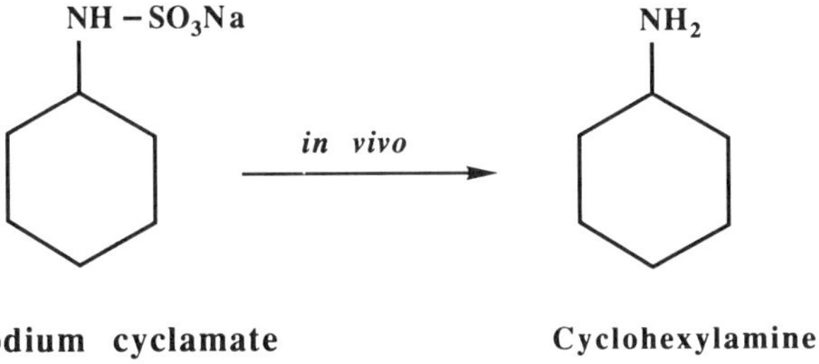

$NH-SO_3Na$ *in vivo* → NH_2

Sodium cyclamate Cyclohexylamine

Figure 9.10 Structures of sodium cyclamate and its metabolite, cyclohexylamine.

from 78 to 105 weeks (except for one earlier death). The *in vivo* conversion from sodium cyclamate to cyclohexylamine was observed particularly in the higher dosage group. Cyclohexylamine is very toxic (LD_{50} rat oral = 157 mg/kg) compared to sodium cyclamate (LD_{50} oral = 12 g/kg). In 1968, the FDA discovered teratogenicity of sodium cyclamate in rats. Its use in food was prohibited in 1969.

V. Coloring Agents

Coloring agents have been used to make food more attractive since ancient times. The perception and acceptability of food is strongly influenced by its color. Both taste and flavor are influenced by color. Nutritionists have long known that without expected color cues, even experts have difficulty in identifying tastes. Certain varieties of commercial oranges have coloring applied to their peels because the natural appearance—green and blotchy—is rejected by consumers as unripe or defective. Consumers reject orange juice unless it is strongly colored, even if

TABLE 9.6
Acute Toxicity of Sodium Cyclamate

Animal	Method	LD_{50} (g/kg)
Mouse	Oral	10–15
Mouse	ip	7
Mouse	Intramuscular injection	4–5
Rat	Oral	12–17
Rat	ip	6
Rat	Intramuscular injection	3–4

it is identical in taste and nutritional value. Congress has twice overridden the FDA (in 1956 and 1959) when it proposed a ban of the coloring agents used.

The natural pigments of many foods are unstable in heat or oxidation. Thus, storage or processing can lead to variations in color even when the nutritional value remains unchanged. Changes in the appearance of a product over time may cause consumers to fear that a "bad" or an adulterated product has been purchased, particularly in light of highly publicized incidents of product tampering. The use of food coloring can resolve this problem for retailers and manufacturers. Ripe olives, sweet potatoes, some sauces, and syrups, as well as other foods, are colored mainly to ensure uniformity and consumer acceptability.

Candies, pastries, and other products such as pharmaceutical preparations are often brightly colored. Pet foods are colored for the benefit of human owners, not their color-blind pets. Such applications are criticized by some as unnecessary, or even frivolous, even when natural food dyes are involved.

Red color can be naturally produced from a dried sugar beet root (beet-red) or from insects such as cochineal (Central America) and lac dye (Southeast Asia). Natural dyes, however, are usually not clear, and their variety is limited. Synthetic coloring agents began to replace them in the late 19th century. Twenty-one synthetic chemicals were recognized for use in 1909 at the Second International Red Cross Conference.

About 80 synthetic dyes were being used in the United States for coloring foods in 1900. At that time, there were no regulations regarding this safety. Many of the same dyes were used to color cloth and only the acute toxicity of these coloring agents was tested before they were used in foods.

The chronology of the addition of new colors is shown in Table 9.7. The number of coloring agents currently permitted as food additives is much fewer than previously and is still being reduced. In 1937, butter yellow (dimethyl amino azobenzene) was found to induce malignant tumors in rats. The carcinogenicity of butter yellow was later confirmed. Then attention began to be directed toward the azo dyes, which contain the azo group (—N=N—) in their structures. There are two kinds of azo dyes, those which are water-soluble and those which are not. In general, the water-soluble azo dyes are less toxic because they are more readily excreted from the body. Either type, however, can be reduced to form the toxic amino group, $—NH_2$, in the body in conjunction with the action of microorganisms such as *Streptococcus, Bacillus pyocyaneus,* and *Proteus* sp. One particular bioassay report on azo compounds showed that only 12 out of 102 azo compounds did not reduce into amine.

TABLE 9.7
Chronology of Newly Developed Synthetic Coloring Agents

Year	Agent
1916	Tartrazine
1918	Yellow AB & OB
1922	Guinea Green
1927	Fast Green
1929	Ponceau SX
1929	Sunset Yellow
1929	Brilliant Blue
1950	Violet No. 1
1966	Orange B
1971	FD&C Red No. 40

A. Amaranth (FD&C Red No. 2)

Amaranth is 1-(4-sulfo-1-naphthylazo)-9-naphthol-3,6-disulfonic acid, trisodium salt (Figure 9.11) and is an azo dye. It is a reddish-brown powder with a water solubility of 12 g/100 ml at 30°C. Before it was prohibited by the FDA in 1976 following indications that it induced malignant tumors in rats, amaranth had been used in almost every processed food with a reddish or brownish color, including soft drinks, ice creams, salad dressings, cereals, cake mixes, wines, jams, chewing gums, chocolate, and coffee as well as a variety of drugs and cosmetics at the level of 0.01–0.0005%. An estimated $2.9 million worth was added in 1973 to more than $10 billion worth of products.

When amaranth (0.5 ml of a 0.1% solution) was injected under the

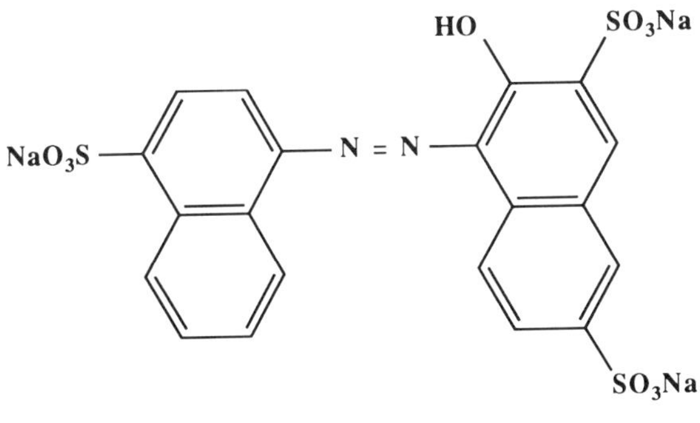

HO SO$_3$Na

NaO$_3$S — N = N —

SO$_3$Na

Figure 9.11 Structure of amaranth.

skin of rats twice a week for 365 days, no tumor growth was observed. When 0.2% of amaranth in feed (average 0.1 g/kg/day) was fed to rats for 417 days, no induction of tumors was observed, but when feeding was continued for an additional 830 days, one case of intestinal cancer was observed. The FAO/WHO special committee determined its ADI as 0–1.5 mg/kg.

Amaranth is metabolized into amine derivatives *in vivo*. Amaranth is reduced by aqueous D-fructose and D-glucose at elevated temperatures to form a mixture of hydrazo and amine species, which may have toxicological significance. The interactions between additives such as amaranth and other food components should be considered from the viewpoint of toxicology.

B. Tartrazine (FD&C Yellow No. 4)

This coloring agent is 5-hydroxy-1-*p*-sulfophenyl-4-(*p*-sulfophenylazo)-pyrazol-3-carboxylic acid, trisodium salt (Figure 9.12). It is a yellow powder and has been used as a food coloring additive since 1916.

The median acute oral lethal dose of tartrazine in mice is 12.17 g/kg. Beagle dogs received tartrazine as 2% of the diet for 2 years without adverse effects, with the possible exception of pyloric gastritis in one dog. Tumor incidence was unchanged relative to controls in rats receiving tartrazine at 1.5% of the diet for 64 weeks and in rats administered this dye at 5.0% of the diet for 2 years.

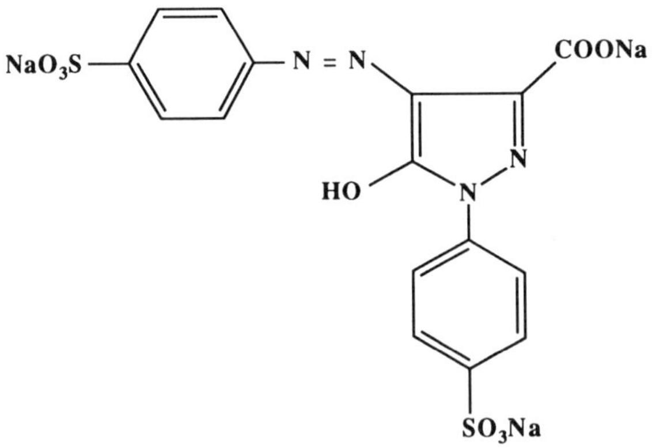

NaO_3S N = N COONa N HO N SO_3Na

Figure 9.12 Structure of tartrazine.

Human sensitivity to tartrazine has been reported with some frequency and has been estimated to occur in 1/10,000 persons. Anaphylactic shock, potentially life-threatening, has been reported but symptoms more commonly cited are urticaria (hives), asthma, and purpura (blue or purple spots on the skin or mucous membrane). Of 97 persons with allergic symptoms in one trial, 32 had adverse reactions to challenge with 50 mg tartrazine. Physicians use 0.1–10 mg tartrazine to test for its sensitivity.

Tartrazine is known as the least toxic coloring agent among synthetic coloring chemicals. In the United States, tartrazine can be used in foods only as a coloring agent (FDA Regulations 8.275, 8.501). Tartrazine is permitted in Great Britain for use as a food-coloring agent. An ADI was set in 1966 at 0–7.5 mg/kg by FDA.

Although many synthetic coloring agents are toxic if used in large enough amounts, and many are suspected carcinogens as well, natural coloring agents are not always safe. Caramel, which gives a light brown color, contains carcinogenic benzo[*a*]pyrene in small amounts; curcumin, which gives the yellow color to curry, is 15 times as toxic as tartrazine.

VI. Flavoring Agents

Flavoring agents increase the acceptability of food. People have long tried to improve the flavor of foods; since the mid-19th century, numerous flavor chemicals have been synthesized. Coumarin was synthesized in 1868; vanilla flavor, vanillin, was synthesized in 1874; cinnamon flavor was made in 1884 (cinnamic aldehyde). By the 20th century, nearly 1000 flavoring chemicals had been developed. At the present time, over 3000 synthetic chemicals are used as flavor ingredients.

As was the case with coloring agents, the toxicity of flavoring agents began to receive attention in the 1960s. Most natural flavors used in the United States are generally recognized as safe (GRAS) on the basis of their occurrence in foods long and widely eaten with no apparent ill effects. These chemicals have been used in large quantities in most food products with little regard for safety. Food industries even attempt to produce flavor ingredient chemicals that are found naturally in plants (so-called natural identical substance). Although it has been assumed that the natural flavorings are not health hazards, there are many toxic

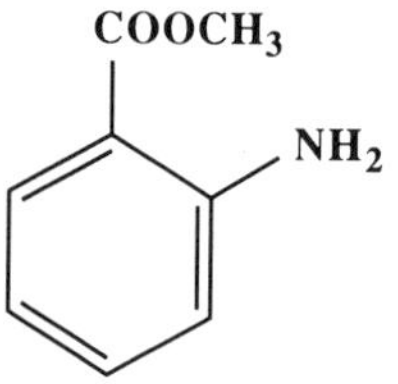

Figure 9.13 Structure of methyl anthranilate.

chemicals in natural products and their chronic toxicity should be carefully reviewed.

A. Methyl Anthranilate

Methyl anthranilate (Figure 9.13) is a colorless liquid which has a sweet, fruity, grape-like flavor. It is found in the essential oils of orange, lemon, and jasmine and has been widely used to create imitation concord grape flavor. Table 9.8 shows the acute toxicity of methyl anthranilate. Methyl anthranilate promotes some allergic reactions on human skin, which has led to it being prohibited for use in cosmetic products.

B. Safrole (3,4-Methylene Dioxallylbenzene)

Safrole (Figure 9.14) is a colorless oily liquid possessing a sweet, warm-spicy flavor. It has been used as a flavoring agent for more than 60 years. Oil of sassafras, which contain 80% safrole, has also been used as a spice. In the United States, the FDA banned the use of safrole in 1958 and many other countries followed this lead and also banned the use of safrole in flavors. Safrole, either that which occurs naturally in sassafras oil or the synthetic chemical, has been shown to induce liver tumors in rats.

TABLE 9.8
Acute Toxicity of Methyl Anthranilate

Animal	LD_{50} (oral, mg/kg)
Mouse	3900
Rat	2910
Guinea pig	2780

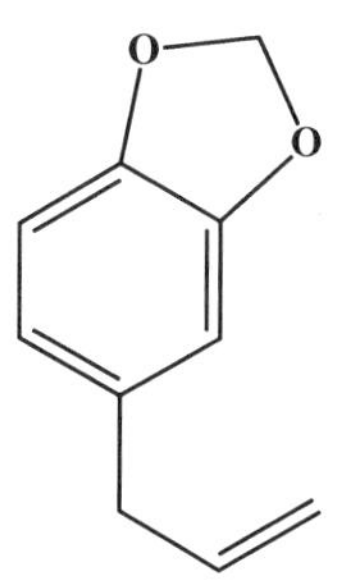

Figure 9.14 Structure of safrole.

VII. Flavor Enhancers

A small number of food additives are used to modify the taste of natural and synthetic flavors even though they do not directly contribute to flavor; such substances are known as flavor enhancers. Most people are familiar with the use of table salt to enhance the flavor of a wide variety of foods. Salt can be an effective enhancer even at levels far below the threshold for salty taste. It is widely used in processed foods such as canned vegetables and soups.

Another well-known enhancer is monosodium glutamate (MSG). Its use as an enhancer has periodically aroused concern about the potential toxicity of a quantity of free glutamate ingested at once. MSG became controversial because of its association with the so-called Chinese Restaurant syndrome. Symptoms of this syndrome, which is usually self-diagnosed, include headache and drowsiness.

Because of these concerns, both the acute and chronic toxicity of MSG have been widely studied. After a review of available data, the FDA affirmed the GRAS status of MSG in the United States. While some individuals are susceptible to transient discomfort following ingestion of MSG, it does not pose any risk of lasting injury.

Suggestions for Further Reading

1. Ayres, J. C., Kirschman, J. C. (ed.) (1981). "Impact of Toxicology on Food Processing." AVI Pub. Co., Westport, Connecticut.
2. Federal Food, Drug, and Cosmetic Act (1971). United States Code, Title 21.
3. Gibson, G. G., and Walker, R. (eds.) (1985). "Food Toxicology: Real or Imaginary Problems? Taylor & Francis, Philadelphia.

4. Gilchrist, A. (1981) "Foodborne Disease and Food Safety." American Medical Association, Monroe, Wisconsin.
5. Hathcock, J. N. (ed.) (1982–1989). "Nutritional Toxicology." Academic Press, New York.
6. Huls, M. E. (1988). "Food Additives and Their Impact on Health." Oryx Press, Phoenix, AZ.
7. Irving, G., Jr. (1982). Determination of the GRAS status of food ingredients. *In* "Nutritional Toxicology" (J. Hathcock, ed.), Vol. I. Academic Press, New York.
8. Lewis, R. J., Sr. (1989). "Food Additives Handbook." Van Nostrand Reinhold, New York.
9. Millstone, E. (1986). "Food Additives." Penguin Books, New York.
10. Office of the Federal Register (1981). Code of Federal Regulations, Title 21, Part 182. United States Government Printing Office, Washington, D.C.
11. Okun, M. (1986). "Fair Play in the Marketplace: The First Battle for Pure Food and Drugs." Northern Illinois University Press, Dekalb, Illinois.
12. Richardson, M. (ed.) (1986). "Toxic Hazard Assessment of Chemicals." Royal Society of Chemistry, London.
13. Ross, K. D. (1975). Reduction of the azo food dyes FD & C Red 2 (Amaranth) and FD & C Red 40 by thermally degraded D-fructrose and D-glucose. *J. Agric. Food Chem.* **23,** 475.

CHAPTER **10**

Toxicants Formed during Food Processing

The development of food processing technology—which includes frying, toasting, roasting, evaporation, smoking, sterilization, pasteurization, irradiation, pickling, freezing, and canning—expanded the potential of food supplies greatly in the modern era. For example, smoke treatment made a year-round supply of fish possible and canned foods could be sent anyplace in the world.

In the United States, commercial food processing is subject to regulation by the FDA and must meet specified standards of cleanliness and safety. Sometimes particular methods of food processing are considered under the category of food additives, since they may intentionally alter the form or nature of food.

Home cooking is one important method of food processing. Cooking increases the palatability (for example, flavor, appearance, texture) and stability of foods; it also improves the digestibility of foods. Moreover, it kills toxic microorganisms and deactivates such toxic substances as enzyme inhibitors. Since antiquity, people appreciated home-cooked food.

The chemical changes in food components, including amino acids, proteins, sugars, carbohydrates, vitamins, and lipids, caused by high-heat treatment have raised questions about the usual consequence of reducing nutritive values and even the formation of some toxic chemicals such as polycyclic aromatic hydrocarbons (PAHs), amino acid or protein pyrolysates, and *N*-nitrosamines. Among the many reactions occurring in processed foods, the Maillard Reaction plays the most important role in the formation of various chemicals (including toxic ones).

During processing, it frequently happens that some foreign materials are mixed into foods. Some of these materials are undesirable ones.

Although most modern food factories are engineered to avoid any occurrence of food contamination during processing, low-level contamination is hard to eliminate entirely. Many instances of accidental contamination of food by toxic materials have been reported. For example, in 1955 in Japan, a neutralizing agent (sodium phosphate) that was contaminated with sodium arsenite was added to milk during a drying process; the final commercial dried milk contained 10–50 ppm of arsenic. Subsequently, many serious cases of arsenic poisoning were reported.

It is a common misunderstanding that gamma irradiation, which is most often used for food irradiation, produces radioactive materials in foods. In fact, although the electromagnetic energy used for irradiation is sufficient to penetrate deep into foods and can kill a wide range of microorganisms, it is far below the range required to produce radioactivity in the target material. However, there are still uncertainties about the toxicity of chemicals that may be produced during irradiation. The energies used are sufficient to produce free radicals, which may in turn produce toxic chemicals.

I. Polycyclic Aromatic Hydrocarbons

Polycyclic aromatic hydrocarbons occur widely in the environment. The typical PAHs are shown in Figure 10.1. They are found in water, soil, dust, and in many foods. For over 200 years, carcinogenic effects have been ascribed to PAHs. In 1775, Percival Pott, an English physician, made the association between the high incidence of scrotal cancer in chimney sweeps and their continual contact with chimney soot. The research on the toxicity of PAHs, however, progressed somewhat slowly. In 1932, benzo[*a*]pyrene (BP) was isolated from coal tar and found to be highly carcinogenic in experimental animals.

A. Occurrence

One of the most abundant food sources of PAHs is vegetable oil. It is possible that the high levels of PAHs in vegetable oils are due to endogenous production, with environmental contamination playing only a minor role. However, some of the PAHs in vegetables are apparently due to environmental contamination because levels of these substances decrease with increased distance from industrialized centers and freeways. The

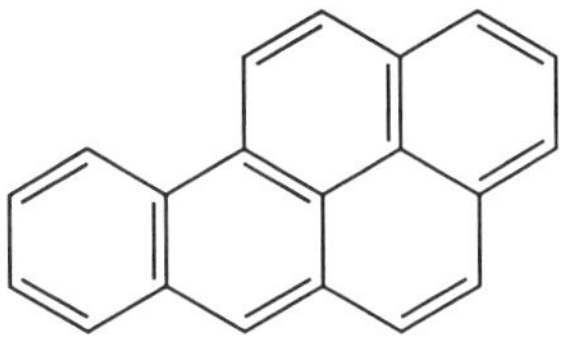

Benzo[a]pyrene

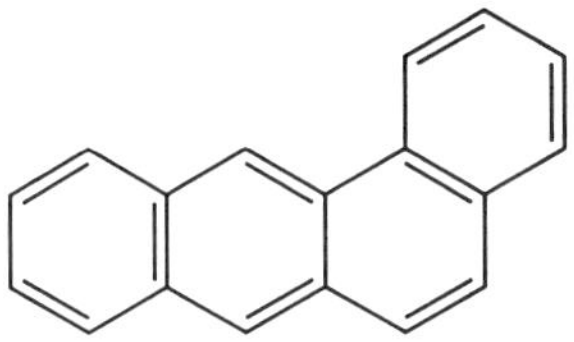

Benzo [a]anthracene

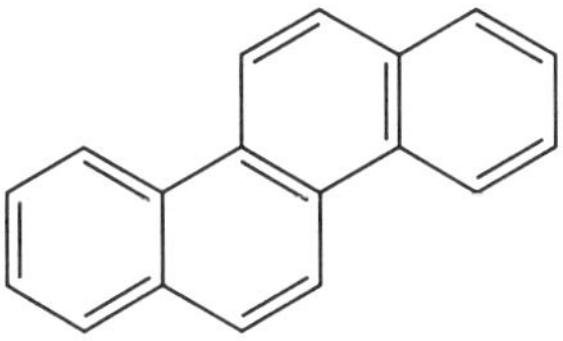

Chrysene

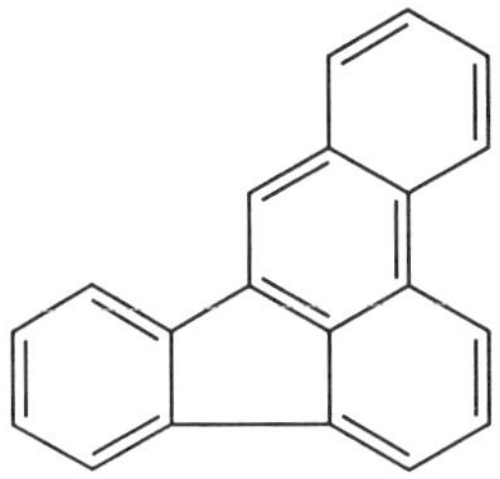

Benzo[b]fluoranthrene

Figure 10.1 Polycyclic aromatic hydrocarbons.

occurrence of PAHs in margarine and mayonnaise appears to be due to contamination of the oils used to make these products.

Levels of PAHs in soil can be quite high, even in areas distant from industrialized centers. Levels of PAHs of 100–200 ppm in the soil were found in some locations distant from human populations. It is thought that these levels result primarily as a residue from decaying vegetation. The significance of these relatively high levels of potentially carcinogenic substances in the soil is not fully understood.

Charcoal broiling or smoking of food also causes PAHs contamination (Table 10.1). PAHs are formed mainly from carbohydrates in foods at high temperatures in the absence of oxygen. Broiling meat over hot ceramic or charcoal briquettes allows the melted fat to come into contact with a very hot surface. PAHs are produced in the ensuing reactions. These products rise with the resulting cooking fumes and are deposited on the meat. Similarly, the presence of PAHs in smoked meats is due to the presence of these substances in smoke. PAHs levels in meat that is cooked at a greater distance from the coals are lower than in meat that is cooked close to the coals. Obviously, food processing produces PAHs in certain levels. It is of major importance to be aware of the presence of carcinogenic PAHs in our foods, and the overall public health hazard should be evaluated and controlled.

TABLE 10.1
Polycyclic Aromatic Hydrocarbons Found in Smoked Foods (ppb)

Food	Benzo[*a*] anthracene	Benzo[*a*] pyrene	Benzo[*e*] pyrene	Fluoranthene	Pyrene
Beef	0.4	—	—	0.6	0.5
Cheese				2.8	2.6
Herring				3.0	2.2
Dried herring	1.7	1.0	1.2	1.8	1.8
Salmon	0.5	—	0.4	3.2	2.0
Sturgeon	—	0.8	—	2.4	4.4
Frankfurters	—	—	—	6.4	3.8
Ham	2.8	3.2	1.2	14.0	11.2

B. Benzo[a]pyrene

The most commonly known carcinogenic PAH is benzo[*a*]pyrene (BP), which is widely distributed in various foods (Table 10.2). BP was reportedly formed at a level of 0.7 and 17 ppb at 370 to 390 and 650°C, respectively, when starch was heated. Amino acids and fatty acids also produced BP upon high-temperature treatment (Table 10.3). Many cooking processes utilize the 370–390°C range; for example, the surface temperature of baking bread may approach 400°C and deep fat frying is 400–600°C, suggesting that cooking produces some PAHs, including BP. The meat inspection division of the USDA and FDA analyzed 60 assorted foodstuffs and related materials for BP. Samples that contain relatively high levels of BP are shown in Table 10.1.

TABLE 10.2
Benzo[a]pyrene Found in Various Foods

Food	Concentration (ppb)
Fresh vegetables	2.85–24.5
Vegetable oil	0.41–1.4
Coffee	0.31–1.3
Tea	3.9
Cooked sausage	12.5–18.8
Smoked hot sausage	0.8
Smoked turkey fat	1.2
Charcoal-broiled steak	0.8
Barbecued ribs	10.5

TABLE 10.3
Amounts of PAHs Produced from Carbohydrates, Amino Acids, and Fatty Acids Heated at 500 and 700°C (μg/50 g)

	Starch		D-Glucose		L-Leucine		Stearic acid	
PAH	500	700	500	700	500	700	500	700
Pyrene	41	965	23	1680	—	1200	0.7	18,700
Fluoranthene	13	790	19	1200	—	320	—	6,590
Benzo[*a*]pyrene	7	179	6	345	—	58	—	4,440

1. *Toxicity*

BP has been subjected to extensive carcinogenic testing. It is a reasonably potent contact carcinogen. Table 10.4 shows the relative carcinogenicity of BP and other PAHs. A diet containing 25 ppm of BP fed for 140 days to mice produced leukemias and lung adenomas in addition to stomach tumors. Skin tumors developed in over 60% of the rats treated topically with approximately 10 mg of benzo[*a*]pyrene three times per week. The incidence of skin tumors dropped to about 20% when treatment was about 3 mg × 3 per week. Above the 10-mg range, however, the incidence of skin tumors increased dramatically to nearly 100%.

The compound is also carcinogenic when administered orally. In one experiment, weekly doses of greater than 10 mg administered for 10 weeks induced stomach cancers, although no stomach cancers were produced at the dose of 10 mg or less. At 100-mg doses, nearly 70% of the animals had developed stomach tumors by the completion of the experiment.

TABLE 10.4
Relative Carcinogenicity of Typical Polycyclic Aromatic Hydrocarbons (PAH)

PAH	Relative activity
Benzo[*a*]pyrene	+ + +[a]
5-Methylchrysene	+ + +
Dibenz[*a,h*]anthracene	+ +
Dibenzo[*a,i*]pyrene	+ +
Benzo[*b*]fluoranthene	+ +
Benz[*a*]anthracene	+
Benzo[*c*]phenanthrene	+
Chrysene	+

[a] + + +, high; + +, moderate; +, weak.

2. *Mode of Toxic Action*

BP is transported across the placenta and produces tumors in the offspring of animals treated during pregnancy. Skin and lung tumors appear to be the primary lesions in the offspring.

The biochemical mechanisms by which benzo[*a*]pyrene initiates cancer have been studied in some detail. Benzo[*a*]pyrene is not mutagenic and carcinogenic by itself, but must be first converted to active metabolites. This metabolic conversion involves initially a cytochrome P450-mediated oxidation, producing a 7,8-epoxide. The 7,8-epoxide, in turn, undergoes an epoxide hydrolase-mediated hydration, producing the 7,8-diol which, upon further oxidation by cytochrome P450, produces the corresponding diolepoxide. This diolepoxide is highly mutagenic without metabolic activation and is also highly carcinogenic at the site of administration. The benzo[*a*]pyrene diolepoxide can react with various components in the cells, including DNA, in which case it is possible that a mutation will occur. This is thought to be the primary event in benzo[*a*]pyrene-induced carcinogenesis.

II. Maillard Reaction Products

In 1912, the French chemist L. C. Maillard hypothesized the reaction that accounts for the brown pigments and polymers produced from the reaction of the amino group of an amino acid and the carbonyl group of a sugar. Maillard also proposed that the reaction between amines and carbonyls was implicated in *in vivo* damages; in fact, the Maillard reaction was later proved to initiate certain damages in biological systems. Some products formed by this reaction in processed foods exhibited strong mutagenicity, suggesting the possible formation of carcinogens.

The summary of the Maillard reaction is shown in Figure 10.2. Many chemicals form from this reaction in addition to the brown pigments and polymers. Because of the large variety of constituents, a mixture obtained from a Maillard reaction shows many different chemical and biological properties: brown color, characteristic roasted or smoky odors, pro- and anti-oxidants, and mutagens and carcinogens, or perhaps anti-mutagens and anti-carcinogens. It is common practice to use the so-called Maillard browning model system consisting of a single sugar and an amino acid to investigate complex, actual, food systems. The results of much mutagenicity testing on the products of Maillard browning model systems have been reported. Some Maillard model systems that produced mutagenic materials are shown in Table 10.5.

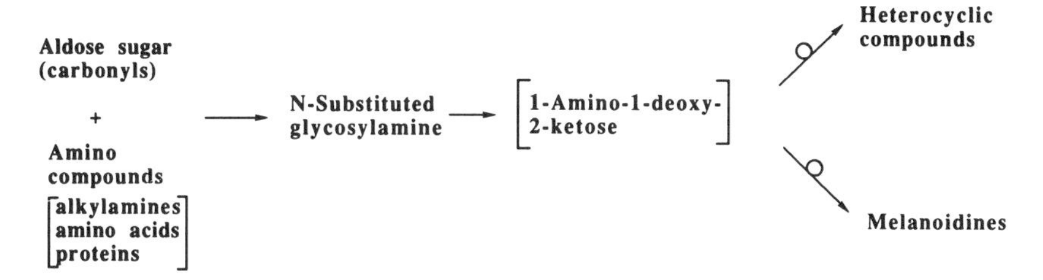

Figure 10.2 Summary of the Maillard reaction.

III. Amino Acid Pyrolysates

In the late 1970s, mutagenicity of pyrolysates obtained from various foods was reported that could not be accounted for by PAHs formed on the charred surface of certain foods such as broiled fish and beef. The mutagenic principles of the tryptophan pyrolysates were later identified as nitrogen-containing heterocyclic compounds. A group of polycyclic aromatic amines is produced primarily during the cooking of protein-rich foods. Their structures are shown in Figure 10.3. The early work on the isolation and production of these substances was based on their mutagenicity. Some classes of cooked protein-rich foods tended to be more

TABLE 10.5
Mutagenic Materials Produced from the Maillard Model System

Model system	*Salmolella typhimurium* strains
D-Glucose/cysteamine	TA 100 without S9[a]
	TA 98 with S9
Cyclotene/NH_3	TA 98 without S9
	TA 1538 without S9
L-Rhamnose/NH_3/H^2S	TA 98 with S9
Maltole/NH_3	TA 98 with S9
	TA 100 with S9
Starch/glycine	TA 98 with S9
Lactose/casein	TA 98 with S9
Potato starch/$(NH_4)_3CO_4$	TA 98 with S9
	TA 100 with S9
Diacetyl/NH_3	TA 98 with S9
	TA 100 with S9

[a] Metabolic activation.

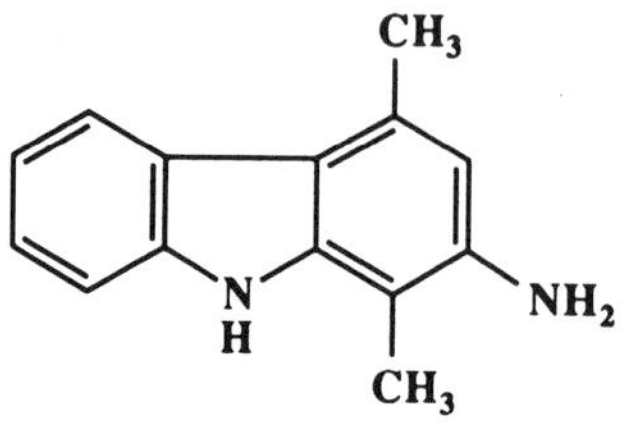

Trp-P-1 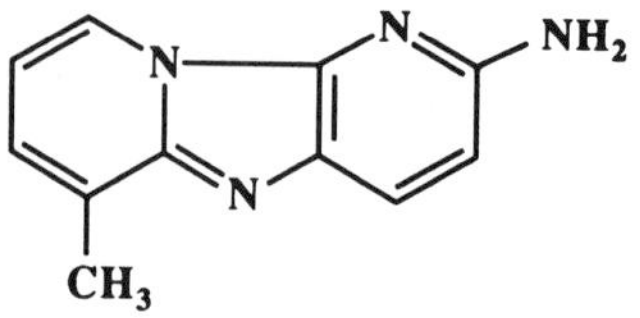 Glu-P-1

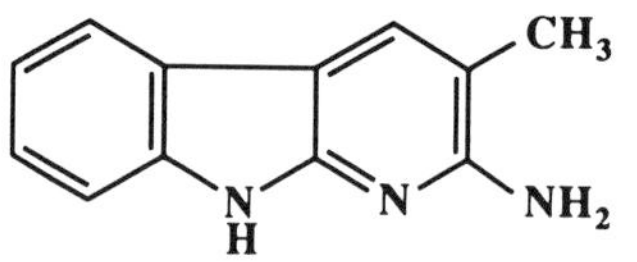

MeAαC 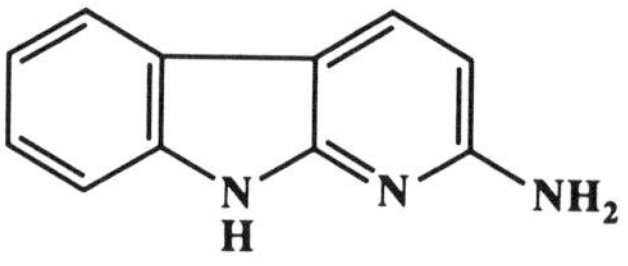 AαC

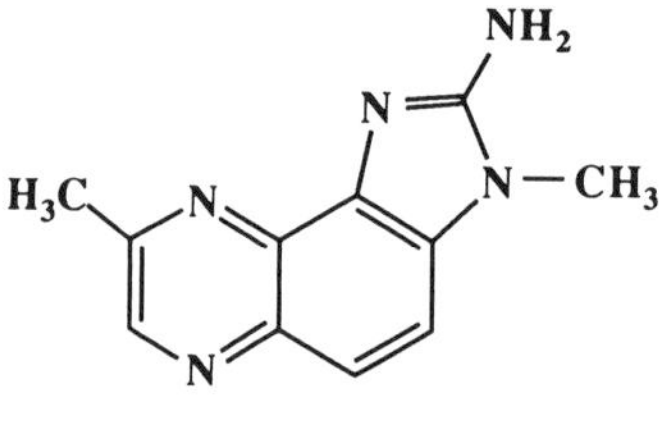

MeIQx 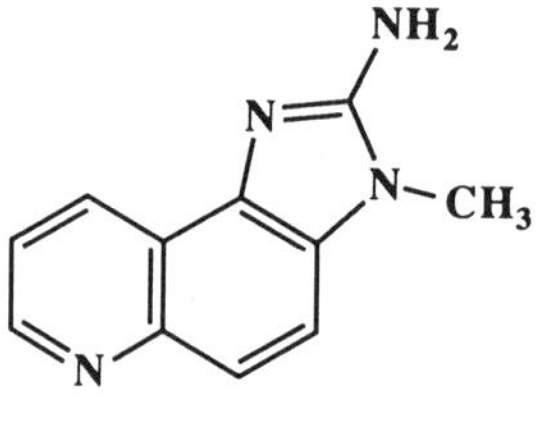 IQ

Figure 10.3 Mutagenic heterocyclic amines.

mutagenic than others, and the extent of heating influenced the level of mutagenic activity. The most highly heated samples of milk, cheese, tofu, rock cod, and several varieties of beans, although heavily charred, were only weakly mutagenic. Hamburger cooked at high temperatures was reported as mutagenic. The mutagenecity was, however, limited to the surface layers where most pyrolysates are found. On the other hand, no mutagenic activity was found in comparable samples of uncooked hamburger meat. The formation of these mutagenic substances seems to depend on temperature, and the temperature dependence of mutagen formation in heated beef stock has been determined quantitatively.

The identities of the mutagens produced under normal cooking conditions have been established in some cases. The major mutagens in broiled fish are the heterocyclic amines imidazoquinoline (IQ) and methylimidazoquinoline (MeIQx) (Figure 10.3). They are also minor components of fried beef. Several other mutagens of this class are also present in cooked meat. Beef extracts, which contain IQ and MeIQx, are metabolically converted to active mutagens by liver tissue from several animal species and humans. Although these substances are highly potent mutagens, they are fairly weak carcinogens in rats. Following the mutagenicity studies on these pyrolysates, carcinogenicity of tryptophane (Trp-P-1 and Trp-P-2) and glutamine (Glu-P-1) were demonstrated using animals such as rats, hamsters, and mice. For example, a high percentage of tumor incidence was observed in mice fed a diet containing Trp-P-1 or Trp-P-2. The various reports indicate that both amino acid and protein pyrolysates may act as carcinogens in the alimentary tracts of experimental animals. Extensive research is presently being conducted to determine whether heterocyclic amines produced during the cooking process are hazardous to humans.

IV. *N*-Nitrosamines

Mixtures of inorganic salts, such as sodium chloride and sodium nitrite, have been used to cure meat for centuries. Only relatively recently has it been recognized that the curing action results from the nitrite ion. Bacterial reduction can produce nitrite from nitrate ions, although today nitrite is used directly. Certain fish products are also cured with nitrite. Some countries (but not the United States) also permit the addition of nitrate in the production of some varieties of cheese.

A. Precursors

1. Nitrite and Nitrate

The nitrite ion plays at least three important roles in the curing of meat. First, it has an antimicrobial action. In particular, it inhibits the growth of the microorganism that produces botulism toxin, *Clostridium botulinum.* The mechanism and cofactors of this antimicrobial action are not understood. However, since cured meats are often stored under anaerobic conditions for extended periods, it is very important in ensuring the safety of these foods. Nitrite also imparts an appealing red color to meats during curing. This color arises from nitrosylmyoglobin and nitrosylhemoglobin pigments. These pigments are formed when nitrite is reduced to nitric oxide, which then reacts with myoglobin and hemoglobin. If these pigments did not form, cured meats would have an unappetizing grayish color. Finally, nitrite gives a desirable "cured" flavor to bacon, frankfurters, ham, and other meat products. The levels of nitrites that are permissible in cured foods vary from country to country and range from 10 to 200 ppm. The major portion of nitrite in humans results from reduction of dietary nitrate by bacteria in the mouth and in the intestinal tract. Nitrate is encountered in the diet, often in relatively high levels (1000–3000 ppm), in vegetables such as cabbage, cauliflower, carrots, celery, and spinach; the levels are variable and the exact causes are uncertain.

Nitrate is widely found in foods. The dietary intake for adult Americans has been estimated at 100 mg per day. Vegetables, especially leaf and root vegetables, account for over 85% of the total, while cured meats contribute about 9%. In certain areas, well water contains high levels of nitrate. While exposure from meat products may have dropped in recent years, the use of nitrate in fertilizers, and its concomitant widespread occurrence in soils and water, means that vegetables continue to be significant sources.

The reduced nitrite is not found in significant amounts in most foods. The chief dietary source is cured meats, in which it is present as an intentional food additive because of its desired antimicrobial, flavor, and color properties. Most ingested nitrite comes from saliva, which is estimated to contribute 8.6 mg of the total daily intake of 11.2 mg from the diet.

B. Occurrence

Nitrosation of secondary and tertiary amines produces stable nitrosamines. Unstable nitroso compounds are produced with primary amines. The reaction rate is pH-dependent and is maximum near pH 3.4. The nitrosation of weakly basic amines is more rapid than that of more strongly basic amines. Several anions, such as halogens and thiocyanate, promote the nitrosation process; on the other hand, antioxidants, such as ascorbate and vitamin E, inhibit the reaction of destroying nitrite. Diethylnitrosamine (DEN) and dimethylnitrosamine (DMN) occur in the gastric juice of experimental animals and humans fed diets containing amines and nitrite. The nitrosation reaction is also known to occur during high-temperature heating of foods, such as bacon, which contain nitrite and certain amines.

In Norway in 1962, following an epidemic of food poisoning in sheep, extremely high levels of nitrosamines were detected in herring meal treated with nitrite as a preservative. The sheep suffered severe liver disease and many of them died. It was later shown that the rate of spontaneous formation of nitrosamine in nitrite-treated fish was dependent on the temperature of preparation following the addition of nitrite. Thus, refrigerated fish treated with nitrite had no more nitrosamine than fresh fish treated with nitrite, but heat treatment of fish increased the rate of nitrosamine formation following addition of nitrite. It was suggested that increased levels of nitrosamines in heated fish are due—at least in part—to increased concentrations of secondary amines resulting from protein degradation during the heating process.

Heating of other nitrite-treated foods has also been shown to produce nitrosamines. Cured meats have all been shown to contain nitrosamines (Table 10.6), the higher levels appearing in cured meats that have been subjected to relatively high heating. It is important to note that the levels of nitrosamines detected in various foods are quite variable. The reasons for this variability are not clear but seem to be dependent on the type of food and the laboratory conducting the examination.

The levels of volatile nitrosamines in spice premixes, such as those used in sausage preparation, were found to be extraordinarily high. These premixes contained spices with secondary amines and a curing mixture that included nitrite. Volatile nitrosamines formed spontaneously in these premixes during long periods of storage. The problem was solved simply by combining the spices and the curing mixture just prior to use.

Analyses of certain beers have also shown considerable variability in levels of nitrosamines. Although the mean concentration of volatile nitrosamines in both American and imported beer is generally quite low, the levels in certain samples can be as high as 70 ppb of dimethylnitrosamine. It was soon found that beers produced from malt dried by direct

TABLE 10.6
Nitrosamine Content in Typical Cured Meats

Meat	Nitrosamine	Level (ppb)
Smoked sausage	Dimethylnitrosamine	< 6
	Diethylnitrosamine	< 6
Frankfurters	Dimethylnitrosamine	11–84
Salami	Dimethylnitrosamine	1–4
Fried bacon	Dimethylnitrosamine	1–40
	Nitrosoproline	1–40

fire rather than by air-drying had the highest levels of nitrosamine. The direct fire-drying process was shown to introduce nitrite into the malting mixture. Domestic beer manufacturers quickly converted to the air-drying process.

C. Toxicity

The carcinogenic activity of many nitrosamines has been examined. Of the over 100 food substances assayed so far, approximately 80% were shown to be carcinogenic in at least one animal species. Diethylnitrosamine is active in 20 animal species. Dimethyl- and diethylnitrosamine are two of the most potent carcinogens in this group. Administration of dimethylnitrosamine at 50 ppm in the diet produces malignant liver tumors in rats in 26–40 weeks. Higher doses produce kidney tumors. As the dose of diethylnitrosamine is reduced below 0.5 mg/kg, the lag period between dosing and onset of tumors increases, with the total tumor yield remaining roughly the same. With a dose of 0.3 mg/kg, the lag time is 500 days, whereas for a dose of 0.075 mg/kg, the lag time is increased to 830 days. No clear threshold dose for carcinogenicity of nitrosamines in the diet has yet been established.

D. Mode of Toxic Action

Nitrosamines, like other groups of chemical carcinogens, require metabolic activation to render them toxic. The activation process is mediated by enzymes and involves, at least in some cases, hydroxylation of the α-carbon (Figure 10.4). The nitrosamines exhibit a good deal of organ specificity in their carcinogenic effect (Table 10.7); for example, dimethylnitrosamine is an active liver carcinogen with some activity in the kidney, and benzylmethylnitrosamine is specific for the esophagus. This organ specificity is apparently due, at least in part, to site-specific metabolism.

Administration of certain nitrosamines to pregnant animals can result in cancer in the offspring. The time of administration seems to be critical. For example, in rats, administration of the carcinogens must occur later than 10 days into gestation to produce cancer in the offspring, and the fetuses are most sensitive just prior to term. This development of sensitivity coincides with the development of the metabolic activation system of the fetuses. In addition, compared to the adults, the fetuses seem to be unusually sensitive to the carcinogenic effects of these substances. For example, at a maternal dose of only 2 mg/kg, which is 2% of

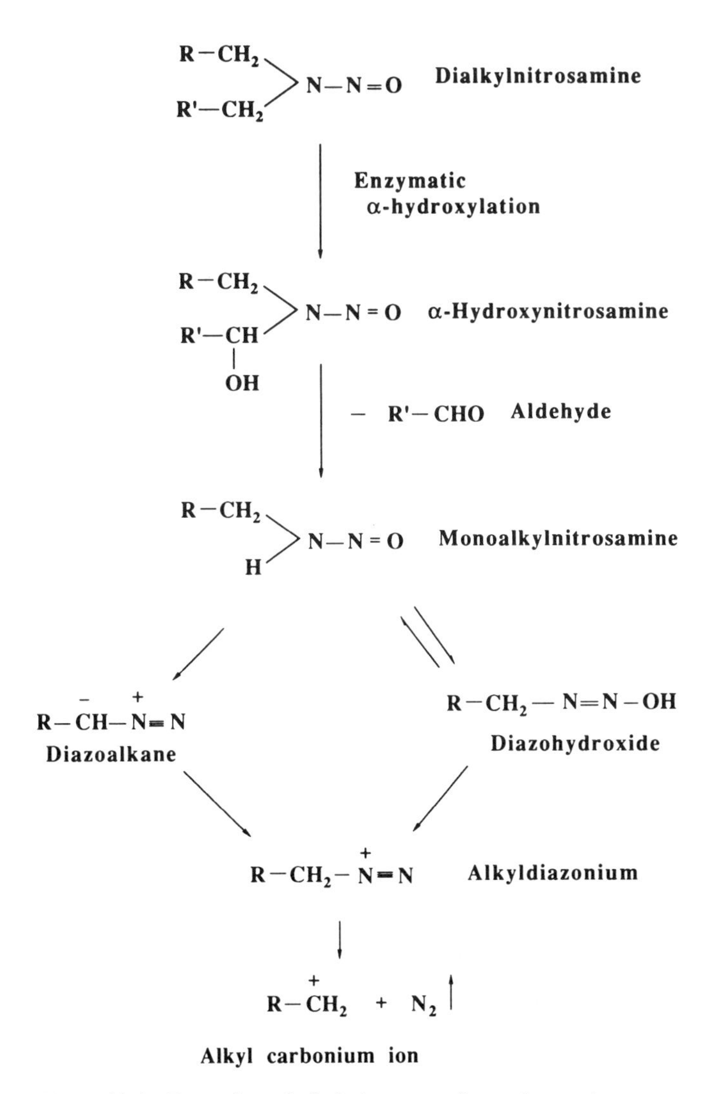

Figure 10.4 Formation of alkylating agent from nitrosamines.

the carcinogenic dose required for adults, N-nitrosoethylurea caused a carcinogenic response in the nervous system of offspring.

Under acidic pH, the nitrite ion can be protonated to form nitrous acid (HONO). The anhydride of nitrous acid, N_2O_3, present in equilibrium with nitrous acid, can nitrosate a variety of compounds, especially secondary and tertiary amines. Halide and thiocyanate ions, present in foods and digestive fluids, can catalyze the formation of *N*-nitroso compounds.

TABLE 10.7
Sites of Tumors Produced by *N*-Nitroso Compounds

Site	Compound
Skin	Methylnitrosourea
Nose	Diethylnitrosamine
Nasal sinus	Dimethylnitrosamine
Tongue	Nitrosohexamethyleneimine
Esophagus	Nitrosoheptamethyleneimine
Stomach	Ethylbutylnitrosamine
Duodenum	Methylnitrosourea
Colon	Cycasin
Lung	Diethylnitrosamine
Bronchi	Diethylnitrosamine
Liver	Dimethylnitrosamine
Pancreas	Nitrosomethylurethane
Kidney	Dimethylnitrosamine
Urinary bladder	Dibutylnitrosamine
Brain	Methylnitrosourea
Spinal cord	Nitrosotrimethylurea
Thymus	Nitrosobutylurea
Lymph nodes	Ethylnitrosourea
Blood vessels	Nitrosomorpholine

E. General Considerations

Efforts to reduce nitrosamine formation in cured meats have been quite successful. Simply adding a reducing agent, such as erythrobate or ascorbate, to the curing mix greatly reduced or eliminated nitrosamine formation in the final product. Domestic manufacturers of cured meat products now generally add these reducing agents to the curing mixture along with the minimum amount of nitrite necessary to achieve the desired effect. However, the nitrosamines found in foods are almost exclusively highly volatile. Very little is presently known about the concentrations of nonvolatile nitrosamines present in foods.

The risk to human health of dietary nitrite and nitrosamines is difficult to assess. As discussed in the preceding section, *in vivo* reduction of the ubiquitous nitrate ion to nitrite appears to be the major source of ingested nitrite, contributing more than three times the nitrite ingested with cured meats in the average American diet. Both catalysts and inhibitors of nitrosation may be present in a typical meal. In addition, there are significant nondietary sources of exposure to nitrosamines and nitrosatable compounds, including tobacco, some pharmaceuticals and cosmetics, and cutting oils used in industry. Isolating effects due to diet alone appears impossible. Nonetheless, it is prudent to minimize controllable exposures.

V. Food Irradiation

In the United States, commercial food processing is subject to regulation by the FDA and must meet specified standards of cleanliness and safety. In certain situations, methods of food processing are considered under the category of food additives since they may intentionally alter the form or nature of food. The use of ionizing radiation to preserve food falls into this category.

Gamma radiation is most often used for food irradiation. Gamma rays are a form of electromagnetic radiation produced by such radioactive elements as Cobalt-60 and Cesium-137. Such sources emit radiation with energies of up to 10 million electron volts (MeV). This is sufficient to penetrate deep into foods, but is far below the range required to produce radioactivity in the target material. Since there is no direct contact between the source and the target, there is no mechanism that can produce radioactivity in irradiated foods.

Studies in the use of ionizing radiation to preserve food began shortly after World War II. A large number of potential applications have been identified. Ionizing radiation can sterilize foods, control microbial spoilage, control insect infestations, and inhibit undesired sprouting. Food irradiation has the potential to substantially reduce postharvest applications of pesticides to prevent spoilage due to insects and fungi. Irradiation can be used to destroy *Salmonella* in cases where heat treatment is not possible, for example, in frozen chicken.

Despite the potential of food irradiation as a preserving technique, it is widely misunderstood and controversial. Some opposition arises from apparent confusion between "irradiated" and "radioactive." Gamma irradiation of foods is in some ways analogous to sterilization of medical equipment with ultraviolet light. Both of these processes can kill a wide range of microorganisms by radiation.

Some other critics have raised questions about the toxicity of chemicals that may be produced during irradiation. The energies used are sufficient to produce free radicals, which can combine with each other or form new bonds to other compounds that may be present. However, it is important to remember that heat treatments commonly used in food processing are likely to produce a higher degree of chemical modification than is irradiation.

Suggestions for Further Reading

1. Ayres, J. C., and Kirschman, J. C. (eds.) (1981). "Impact of Toxicology on Food Processing." AVI Publishing Co., Westport Connecticut.
2. Diehl, J. F., (1990). "Safety of Irradiated Foods." Marcel Dekker, New York.
3. Doyle, J. (1985). "Altered Harvest: Agriculture, Genetics, and The Fate of The World's Food Supply." Viking, New York.
4. Hathcock, J. N. (ed.) (1982–1989). "Nutritional Toxicology." Academic Press, San Diego.
5. Miller, E. C., Miller, J. A., Hirono, I., Sugimura, T., and Takayama, S. (eds) (1979). "Naturally Occurring Carcinogens, Mutagens, and Modulators of Carcinogenesis." University Park Press, Baltimore.
6. Okun, M. (1986). "Fair Play in the Marketplace: The First Battle for Pure Food and Drugs." Northern Illinois University Press, Dekalb, Illinois.
7. Ory, R. L. (ed.) (1981). "Antinutrients and Natural Toxicants in Foods." Food & Nutrition Press, Westport, Connecticut.
8. Board on Toxicology and Environmental Health Hazards, Commission on Life Sciences (1983). "Polycyclic Aromatic Hydrocarbons: Evaluation of Sources and Effects." Committee on Pyrene and Selected Analogues. National Academy Press, Washington, D.C.
9. Roberts, H. R. (ed.) (1981). "Food Safety." Wiley, New York.
10. Urbain, W. M. (1986). "Food Irradiation." Academic Press, Orlando.
11. Webb, T., and Lang, T. (1987). "Food Irradiation: The Facts." Thorsons, Rochester, Vermont.

Index

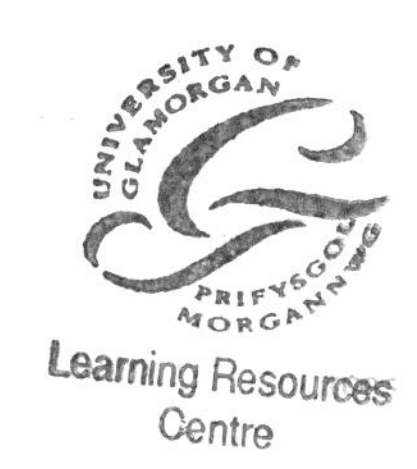

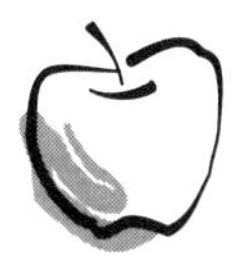

FOOD SCIENCE AND TECHNOLOGY

International Series

Maynard A. Amerine, Rose Marie Pangborn, and Edward B. Roessler, *Principles of Sensory Evaluation of Food.* 1965.

Martin Glicksman, *Gum Technology in the Food Industry.* 1970.

C. R. Stumbo, *Thermobacteriology in Food Processing,* second edition. 1973.

Aaron M. Altschul (ed.), *New Protein Foods:* Volume 1, *Technology,* Part A—1974. Volume 2, *Technology,* Part B—1976. Volume 3, *Animal Protein Supplies,* Part A—1978. Volume 4, *Animal Protein Supplies,* Part B—1981. Volume 5, *Seed Storage Proteins*—1985.

S. A. Goldblith, L. Rey, and W. W. Rothmayr, *Freeze Drying and Advanced Food Technology.* 1975.

R. B. Duckworth (ed.), *Water Relations of Food.* 1975.

John A. Troller and J. H. B. Christian, *Water Activity and Food.* 1978.

A. E. Bender, *Food Processing and Nutrition.* 1978.

D. R. Osborne and P. Voogt, *The Analysis of Nutrients in Foods.* 1978.

Marcel Loncin and R. L. Merson, *Food Engineering: Principles and Selected Applications.* 1979.

J. G. Vaughan (ed.), *Food Microscopy.* 1979.

J. R. A. Pollock (ed.), *Brewing Science,* Volume 1—1979. Volume 2—1980. Volume 3—1987.

J. Christopher Bauernfeind (ed.), *Carotenoids as Colorants and Vitamin A Precursors: Technological and Nutritional Applications.* 1981.

Pericles Markakis (ed.), *Anthocyanins as Food Colors.* 1982.

George F. Stewart and Maynard A. Amerine (eds.), *Introduction to Food Science and Technology,* second edition. 1982.

Malcolm C. Bourne, *Food Texture and Viscosity: Concept and Measurement.* 1982.

Héctor A. Iglesias and Jorge Chirife, *Handbook of Food Isotherms: Water Sorption Parameters for Food and Food Components.* 1982.

Colin Dennis (ed.), *Post-Harvest Pathology of Fruits and Vegetables.* 1983.

P. J. Barnes (ed.), *Lipids in Cereal Technology.* 1983.

David Pimentel and Carl W. Hall (eds.), *Food and Energy Resources.* 1984.

Joe M. Regenstein and Carrie E. Regenstein, *Food Protein Chemistry: An Introduction for Food Scientists.* 1984.

Maximo C. Gacula, Jr., and Jagbir Singh, *Statistical Methods in Food and Consumer Research.* 1984.
Fergus M. Clydesdale and Kathryn L. Wiemer (eds.), *Iron Fortification of Foods.* 1985.
Robert V. Decareau, *Microwaves in the Food Processing Industry.* 1985.
S. M. Herschdoerfer (ed.), *Quality Control in the Food Industry,* second edition. Volume 1—1985. Volume 2—1985. Volume 3—1986. Volume 4—1987.
Walter M. Urbain, *Food Irradiation.* 1986.
Peter J. Bechtel (ed.), *Muscle as Food.* 1986.
H. W.-S. Chan (ed.), *Autoxidation of Unsaturated Lipids.* 1986.
F. E. Cunningham and N. A. Cox (eds.), *Microbiology of Poultry Meat Products.* 1987.
Chester O. McCorkle, Jr. (ed.), *Economics of Food Processing in the United States.* 1987.
J. Solms, D. A. Booth, R. M. Dangborn, and O. Raunhardt, *Food Acceptance and Nutrition.* 1987.
Jethro Jagtiani, Harvey T. Chan, Jr., and Williams S. Sakai (eds.), *Tropical Fruit Processing,* 1988.
R. Macrae (ed.), *HPLC in Food Analysis,* second edition. 1988.
A. M. Pearson and R. B. Young, *Muscle and Meat Biochemistry.* 1989.
Dean O. Cliver (ed.), *Foodborne Diseases.* 1990.
Majorie P. Penfield and Ada Marie Campbell, *Experimental Food Science,* third edition. 1990.
Leroy C. Blankenship (ed.), *Colonization Control of Human Bacterial Enteropathogens in Poultry.* 1991.
Yeshajahu Pomeranz, *Functional Properties of Food Components,* second edition. 1991
Reginald H. Walter (ed.), *The Chemistry and Technology of Pectin.* 1991.
Herbert Stone and Joel L. Sidel, *Sensory Evaluation Practices,* second edition. 1993.
Robert L. Shewfelt and Stanley E. Prussia (eds.), *Postharvest Handling: A Systems Approach.* 1993.
R. Paul Singh and Dennis R. Heldman, *Introduction to Food Engineering,* second edition. 1993.
Tilak Nagodawithana and Gerald Reed (eds.), *Enzymes in Food Processing,* third edition. 1993.
Takayaki Shibamoto and Leonard Bjeldanes, *Introduction to Food Toxicology.* 1993.
Dallas G. Hoover and Larry R. Steenson (eds.), *Bacteriocins of Lactic Acid Bacteria.* 1993.
John A. Troller, *Sanitation in Food Processing,* second edition. 1993
Ronald S. Jackson, Wine Science: *Principles and Applications.* In Preparation.
Robert G. Jensen and Marvin P. Thompson (eds.), *Handbook of Milk Composition.* In Preparation.
Tom Brody, *Nutritional Biochemistry.* In Preparation.